"Your PureLifestyle Plan"

Permanent Weight Loss & Simple Steps to Nutritional Literacy

By Dr.Isabel @ PureLifestyle

Table of Contents <><><><>

International Edition, 2012

First Published in 2012

Introduction: <><><><>

"If you don't like it, change it."

-Unknown

I have been a doctor since 1991, and the only reason I went into the medical field is because I wanted to help people. Looking at what is going on in medicine today, I have come to the realization that, we do not have a Healthcare System, we have Disease Management. Not only did I become disillusioned and burnt out, I just got frustrated treating conditions, not the cause of the problem. My goal is to see people healed.

I wanted to get to the root of the dis-ease. Not just throw a band-aid on it. My patients weren't getting any better, they were just existing.

Hence the reason for the above quotation ..."If you don't like it, change it." I had to change the way I was doing medicine, and let me say it is not easy. But I knew I had to do it for the people I care for, and my sanity.

Over the last decade I began to learn about nutrition, exercise, and lifestyle choices to help you live a more healthy life. Yes, I want to help make a positive change in your life. My goal is to add value to your life, by depositing simple back pocket principles that you can use everyday.

If you want to lose weight permanently, have more energy and infect the lives of your family and friends with health, then I welcome you to "Your PureLifestyle Way".

Congratulations on purchasing *Your PureLifestyle Way!*

Becoming a Registered Reader: <><><><>

Over the next few years, we will be experiencing a revolution in Medicine, and we are all invited. Where everyone will be given the tools to have better health, and not have to live with chronic un-wellness.

Because you have invested in your health by purchasing this book, we would like to keep you up to date with the latest nutritional information. To do so we ask that you become a registered reader and send your email to :

info@doctorisabel.co.nz

Check www.doctorisabel.co.nz for the upcoming date of "Your PureLifestyle Cleanse" for your start to permanent weight loss.

Dedication: <><><><>

I want to dedicate this book to two very special people in my life.

To Mima (aka Mom, Silvia): Your beautiful love and faith in me I will never, ever forget.

To my husband, Michael: Your devoted, love, patience, and maximizing friendship steered me while I said, "Let's go this way."

Opening Quote: <><><><>

"Within every patient, there resides a doctor, and we as physicians are at our best when we put our patients in touch with the doctor inside themselves."

- Albert Schweitzer M.D.

Success Stories: <><><><>

#1. Attending "Your PureLifestyle Plan" gave Murray and I the impetus to make several big but necessary changes to our lifestyle. The course was presented in a fun interactive way and gave us the motivation to make some healthy changes. Before attending the course we had often talked about making some changes but had never got around to it or even where to start. Since doing the course we have built regular exercise routine and big changes in our eating habits. Thanks Mike and Izzy! We would definately recommend this course to anyone who is thinking they could do with a healthier lifestyle. The benefits are well worth it.

Murray and Vicki Crozier.

#2. I chose to take part in "Your PureLifestyle Plan" for a number of reasons, but most of all because I knew the way I was living, eating and thinking was not going to see me through life in good health, after all take-aways and rubbish food are so convenient not to mention life is so busy that we all forget that we still need to find a balance.

Throughout the course I was blessed to be given the tools that would ensure to see me through life not only as a healthy individual but also to be able to hand down those tools to family, friends and the wider community. These tools include healthy cooking and eating, which foods are going to cause illness and damage to my precious body, how to exercise without having the excuse of "I don't have time" as well as how important it is to have a happy healthy brain that can plant positive seeds to grow a positive person.

Since completing the course my health and outlook on life has completely changed with such awesome results, thanks to the tools "Your PureLifestyle Plan" provided me with we as a family now live a healthy active and fun filled life and not once has it been a struggle to implement this into our day to day living. I cannot Thank Mike and Izzy enough for saving me and my family from the convenience and fuss of today's busy lifestyles. Mike and DR Izzy, you guys rock; Thanks, Nita Gaylord

#3. Hi my name is Heather Valdez, I just want to say a few words about my experience of attending "PureLifestyle Plan". Earlier this year myself and three of my children attended the Peak Energy For Life program. Michael and Doctor Isabel Hunsinger presented an extremely enjoyable and informative program. This couple are truly passionate and knowledgeable about health and living a healthy life style. Michael being an experienced Executive Chief and Isabel a Doctor, you could not ask for better teachers to deliver this life changing program.

I learned so much from Isabel about how the body works. Why we feel tired after eating certain foods, hungry not long after you have just eaten. The good foods we can eat that give us energy and we stay full for longer. One of the best things I enjoyed was learning how to loose weight without that nasty four letter work "DIET." Eat, not go hungry and loose weight. Learning how the body works, why it does what it does and why your energy levels feel they way they do, was amazing to learn. The way Isabel presented the information made it fun and easy to learn. You can feel her passion.

Once we learnt about the different foods we had a cooking night with "Executive Chief Mike." WOW, PRICELESS. Are two words I have to say about what I came away with that night. Mike made it so easy to make a healthy meal and incorporate 9 -12 different colour fruits and vegetables in a meal. I am a mother who works a full time career. I use to always stress over what to make for dinner in a timely manner, so the children would still get to bed on time.

Mike showed us how to spend a couple of hours once a week cutting up your veges, how to keep them fresh in the refrigerator. Prepare your meat for the week. Open your fridge and everything is there that you need to cook healthy meals for the week. I now know how to make healthy meals in a little amount of time for my family. That for me is priceless. I just want to thank Chef Michael and Dr. Isabel from the bottom of my heart for putting together such an amazing, life changing program. I have learnt so much and for that I thank you.

My Story: <><><><>

I was born on Dec. 26 1959 in Washington DC. Now I don't tell everyone my birthday, however because you have decided to read this, I thought it best that you get to know how I became a doctor.

The decision to become a doctor was planted in my mind when I was 5 years old. My uncle, who was an anaesthesiologist, Dr. Julio Perez, has this amazing way about him. When he would walk into the room his smile, his positive attitude, would light up the room. He would just make you feel happy, and you would start smiling.

It was at 5 years of age that I decided, and said to my mom, "I want to be a doctor like Tio Julito (uncle Julio in spanish)"

At 18 , after graduating from high school I was looking through a Mother Earth Magazine and saw that there was an organic farm in Pennsylvania that needed help. A few weeks later I was working at the Lefevers Organic Farm in Spring Grove Pa. That was an eye opening expierence. Not only did I learn how to grow our own sprouts on the windowsill of the kitchen, but was exposed to mulching, running a health food shop, and organic farming.

Winter came and there was no work at the farm, and I was referred to two ladies that were opening a Health Food Restaurant in York Pa., called The Sproutery. The owners Paula and Cindy were really into fresh vegetable juices and I was the "Juicer girl". We were juicing wheatgrass, carrot, celery, and beetroot, by the glass. It was new, fun, and exciting.

In 1979 I decided It was time to get serious and go to college. After all the exposure to organic farming and eating, I naturally decided to major in Agriculture and become an Organic Farmer. I thought Colorado would be a good place ,so I applied to Colorado State University (CSU), got an interview, and hopped on a bus with my 3 liter bottle of organic apple juice and fasted the whole way (3 days to be exact) until I was deposited in the Fort Collins, Colorado, bus depot.

The acceptance letter came in the mail and I was off to CSU to become an organic farmer.

There was just one little problem I encountered in my first year of college.....I soon realized that plants don't talk to you and I am a very social being. So, I decided again that I was going to become a doctor.

I withdrew from Agriculture and headed to Boulder Colorado to start my new major, this time as a pre-med student in Molecular Cellular Developmental Biology. I absolutely loved-loved-loved this major, because it taught me how everything works from the DNA level, all the way to the completed picture of the human being.

During the middle of the 4 year degree I was having thoughts of becoming a naturopath. The rationale was it was more holistic and I would learn about taking care of the root of the disease. I really wanted to take care of people without drugs. I mentioned this to my anatomy professor Dr.Tom Swain. He shook his head, smiled that gorgeous smile that he always had, and recommended for me to go the MD way. His philosophy was, you can make more change in medicine once you are on the inside as an MD. He knew I was already unhappy with the medical system for its lack of treating the root cause of the disease, and instead, treat it with medication. I wasn't even a doctor yet, I was still in pre-med....but I knew I needed to become a doctor.

There are times in my life that I become pensive and wonder what my life would have been like if I would have become rebellious and prideful and not taken Dr. Swain's advice. To this date, I am so grateful he cared enough to mentor me into medicine. Thank you Tom.

I made it through medical school and found it very unfair and cutthroat. The amount of minutia we had to memorize seemed and still seems pointless. The whole system would benefit with an overhaul.

After 22 years of being a doctor now I have seen my patients become more unwell and more overweight. They just aren't getting any better. So over the last 10 years I have been studying Functional Medicine, which focuses on the root cause of disease and its treatments. One passion of mine is weight loss because I know how distressful even an extra 5 pounds (2.2 kg) can be, let alone 100 pounds (45 kgs).

Let me give you and overview of my previous health. During my medical training a typical breakfast was a packet of skittles and coffee. Then throughout the day just to stay awake I would have at least 6 cups of coffee . When there was time I would eat a meal. Then when work was done and I didn't have to sleep in the hospital, I would go home. To me 5 o'clock meant wine o'clock, and I would have a glass or two to wind down from all the caffeine.

Not only was I hooked on caffeine and sugar, but also a nighttime wine to wind down. I also partook in cigarette smoking. Yes, I was a model child for health. It took me 41 times to quit smoking but I finally did it. From that comes my motto to my patients " Never, ever, ever give up, Giving up!"

With my second child, I went into the hospital weighing in at 198 pounds (90 kg) and came out at 189 pounds. I am only 5 feet 6 inches (166cm) ! It took me 16 years to get down to 160 pounds (73 Kg) and I did every diet possible except take diet pills. I was deeeeeesperate. Now over the last 2 years, from all my studying, I am 61 kg (135 lbs) at 53 years young and I am so excited to share with you how to get rid of excess weight safely and keep it off.

My conversion to the other side of the medical spectrum happened gradually, and hit it's stride when I had my 50th birthday. I just realized that I really wanted to be healthy and walk my talk. And so here we are together. Let's start walking together, and I'll share with you what worked for me and can also work for you. I want to give you hope.

Your friend; Dr.Isabel

"Hope is not pretending that problems don't exist. It is the hope that they don't last forever. That hurts will heal and difficulties overcome. That we will be led out of the darkness and into the light".

-The Optimism Revolution

Part One: Your Metabolism and Your Nutrition;
People are destroyed by Lack of Knowledge <><><><>

Ch.1 The Circle of Change...Ouch!

Why, do we do what we do, when we know, what we know? That is the question we need to ask ourselves when we are deciding to make a change. For instance, we know smoking is not good for your health, however people continue to smoke. Yes it has to do with the addiction, and it also has a lot to do with the circle of change.

The circle of change pertains to the doors we go through as we are changing. No one likes to change. It feels uncomfortable. We have set habits in place and even if they are killing us, they ARE familiar to you. They bring a sense of stability to our lives.

There are two human tendencies, we as individuals, seek. We either avoid pain or seek pleasure. Which one do you think wins? Yes, you are right ...Avoidance of Pain. We will do anything to avoid pain.

The avoidance of pain is why everyone, including me, wants a quick fix. A quick fix to weight loss. The reality is, there will never be a quick fix. There is no such thing as microwaveable health. We have to put in the work to get the results. The cool thing is that what you will learn here in Your PureLifestyle Plan how to create new, healthy habits that will keep the weight off .

You will create a "New Normal " for yourself. And when you fall off track, as we all do, you will notice that you feel wrong. Heather Valdez, one of my clients in New Zealand says it best, "When I fall off track and start eating the wrong foods...I feel dirty and want to get clean again." That is exactly the point, Heather has created a "New Normal" for herself and it is comfortable for her.

Let's take a look at the phases you go through to create change.

Phase 1. Pre-contemplation; This is called the waiting game. The door is shut tight. This is, as a healthcare worker, the most frustrating stage for me. Why? Because I am waiting for people to either wake up, or just be pushed into having to change their situation. For instance, imagine its 8am in the morning and you are getting ready for work, and on the way to work, bam you start having chest pain. You next are in the Emergency department being told you are having a heart attack. This could be the time you are pushed into doing something about your health or maybe not.

However, if you do start to think about making some lifestyle change then you are moving into the next phase.

Phase 2. Contemplation. The door is slightly ajar. This is when you are thinking about making a change. It is here you start to build your confidence. You are looking at ways to "make the change" as Michael Jackson says.

Phase 3. Preparation. I love this phase because the door is open and it's time for intervention. You are teachable and motivated.

Phase 4. Action and Maintenance Stage. Here you are managing your craving by controlling your challenging thoughts. When problems arise you have a plan of attack.

Phase 5a. The goal is reached. Here you either reset a new goal or stay at your new level for normal.

or

Phase 5b. The relapse and we are back at phase 1. This is where we wait for phase 2 to begin.

So now you know why people do what they do, when they know what they know. It all goes back to where they are in the circle of change.

I trust you are all in phase 3. And for reaching this phase; Let me be the first to tell you today, if no one has beat me to it already, that you are a radiant being!

I cannot change you or anyone. You come to this stage all on your own. In the past I use to push people to this stage and it was like pushing a parked car uphill. Nothing happened.

I learned along time ago that, you can lead a horse to water, HOWEVER if that horse does not want to drink...guess what? It won't.

If you change and achieve your goal because of something I taught you, then all the applause goes to you. You have made the decision to change and implement what you have learned. I didn't change you, you did. You made the decision for a better life with better health. You own that power, not me. Yes, you are truly a radiant being.

About writing down your goals.

Studies have shown that people who write down their goals have a higher rate of achieving them then people who don't. By doing so, the launch begins and the next step appears. If you don't then the next execution step does not appear.

"But what if I don't reach my goal?" That is a fantastic question. No big deal, you reset it. At least you started moving forward and up.

Before we go any further, as your health coach, I ask you to write down the following:

1. What is your goal?

2. Why? Why do care about your health? It's a domino affect.

I'll give you an example. For me, I have pictures of my family in my mind. They need me to be my best for the journey. My husband Michael says "Happy wife, happy life." That is certainly true and I have a responsibility to do my part to make a "happy wife, mother, doctor, friend."

I also think of my goals in life. In particular, my goal in medicine is to coach more than a million health workers around the world. From there, they then go into schools, business's, families, places of worship to purchase back their health, both mentally and physically

3. What would stop you or detour you from reaching your goal? Is it your family, friends, work mates? Ok, its good to know where the bumps in the road will be so you can be prepared.

4. Who is on your support team? TEAM stands for together everyone achieves more. You know I am on your team, but who else? You need to be on your team and be kind to yourself when you are talking to yourself.

Remember that what you conceive, you can achieve. By writing your goals down you are conceiving.

Now that you have that completed, we can go onto the next step. I encourage you to take the time to invest into yourself by writing #1-4 down.

Ch.2 Blood sugars:

What we eat and when we eat affects our energy levels. Until recently, we have been told to eat a low fat diet. This recommendation came into affect in the 1980's. As a result, anyone who wanted to lose weight started to eat anything that said low-fat.

We have been doing that now for 3 decades and how is it going? Are we a more trim and healthy nation? No. We are more overweight and the tsunami of diabetes is hitting our shores. Type 2 Diabetes is a lifestyle disease. It is based on our lifestyle habits and what we eat.

The health industry and the food industry have encouraged us to "take personal responsibility" for our health. If we are overweight it is our fault. We need to watch what we eat and exercise more. I no longer blame anyone for being overweight after I was re-educated about our food.

Our fast food industry is creating fake foods that are so addictive that people just go back for more like a cocaine addict goes back for their next fix. Think about the man in the movie called "Supersize Me". He made a commitment to eat fast foods for 30 days. The first few days he was vomiting after the meals, like a teenage who drank to much. Then towards the end, his cholesterol increased and he gain 30 pounds. What is most important is he felt depressed, tired, and irritable if he didn't go and eat another super sized fast food meal. What happened? He became addicted to the junk food.

David Kessler MD, the former head of the Food and Drug, wrote about this in The End of Overeating. In it he describes the science of how food is made into drugs by creation of hyper-palatable foods that lead to chemical addictions. People are becoming addicted to junk food and we are getting bigger and sicker.

On the flip side people say, "no, you still have to take personal responsibility for being fat." Well then what do we say about a 3 year old that is obese. What personal responsibility does that child need to exert? They are fat because of the foods they are given. If this child lives in a food desert, which are predominant in poor neighborhoods, which lack fresh fruit and vegetable stores, then they are at more risk of obesity.

I have been addicted to French fries and hamburgers in the past but I got some education under my belt and decided to take back my health. My desire is to lay the basic nutrition foundation for you to build on.

Next we will talk about your blood sugar levels. Research shows that low blood sugar levels are associated with lower overall blood flow to the brain, which means more bad decisions. Let's take a look at the graph below to understand why we eat after certain foods.

Our blood sugar levels are affected by what we eat. Our body tells us when we are hungry based on our blood sugar levels. Our body's goal is to keep our blood sugars at a certain level. If it falls to low then a message is sent to eat food.

Eating Carbohydrates

When we eat a carbohydrate, for instance a piece of toast. Our blood sugar spikes, and by 60-90 minutes, our blood sugar is low and we need to eat again. That's why when our kids are drinking an energy drink, which has about 7-13 teaspoons of sugar per drink, and a piece of toast or cereal for breakfast, they will be looking for food in 60-90 minutes. They have just eaten carbohydrates.

I am not saying not to eat carbs. Carbohydrates are very important for our wellbeing. However the right carbohydrates are more important.

Another point to keep in mind is this. When we eat carbs, insulin, a hormone release from the pancreas is released. The carbohydrate spike stimulates insulin which has one major purpose and that is to store excess sugar as fat. Insulin will store fat anywhere. Insulin particularly loves to store fat as Belly Fat.

Eating Carbohydrate + Protein

Now we add a protein such as egg with our toast. This equates with us not being hungry for at least 2.5 - 3 hours. As you can see there is less of a spike in our blood sugar level, which results in less insulin release. The less insulin spike, the less belly fat.

Eating Carbohydrate + Protein + Fat

Now we add some butter to our toast. Our blood sugar levels extend further and do not start dropping until 3.5-4 hours. So we won't start looking for more food to eat to get our blood sugar levels up.

Take a look at the insulin level when you eat a carb + protein + fat. Here we see less of an insulin spike therefore less insulin released which results in less belly fat! Isn't the body amazing.

In summary, the reason we see so much obesity has a lot to do with the fact that people are just eating only carbohydrates. After about an hour they are hungry again because their blood sugars are going down and their bodies are screaming ," Find me more food ". We are very obedient and go to the fastest form of food for the fastest form of energy. Then insulin spikes, and there you have it ...more belly fat.

What are carbohydrates, proteins and fats?

Carbohydrates

- Flour such as bread scones biscuits, pastries and pasta

- Sugar; candy or lolli's, honey , jam etc.

- Legumes; kidney beans, chickpeas, baked beans, black beans

- Potatoes, sweet potatoes, kumara, pumpkin, taro, parsnips

- Veggies and fruit as in corn, peas, bananas, watermelon, pineapple

- Beer, wine, spirits

- Fruit juice and energy drinks

Proteins

- Meat; pork , lamb, chicken, beef

- Fish; tuna, salmon etc.

- Eggs

- Dairy ; yoghurt (plain), cheese, cottage cheese, cream cheese

- Tofu

- Nuts; peanuts, almonds, cashews, walnuts, macadamia

- Seeds; pumpkin, sesame, chia seeds

Fats

- Fat on meat

- Chicken skin

- Lard

- Butter

- margarine

- Oil; coconut oil, olive oil, canola oil, sesame oil etc.

- Salad dressings

- Mayonnaise

   Now you have the basics of what constitutes a carbohydrate, protein and fat. What you want to achieve is to have all three of these every 3-4 hours to keep your blood sugars stable. By doing so, you won't have sharp blood sugar spikes, which makes insulin spike which results in belly fat accumulation.

At www.doctorisabel.co.nz, you can print the FREE Dr.Isabel Food Pyramid, which you can use to guide you on your food choices throughout the day.

People find it easy to use. Pay particular attention to the foundation of the pyramid. It consists of 5-6 servings of vegetables and 1-2 servings of fruit per day. Everyday is the goal.

Taking back your health is much like remodeling your home. You can redecorate every room but the cracks in the floors and walls (the foundation) will just keep sagging until eventually it collapses. If you get the foundation right , the rest will stand and endure. When storms come the home will still be standing.

This is just like life. When the storms of life come you will be able to go through and come out standing.

Ch.3 Why and How Body Stores Fat.

The reason why our body stores fat is to have a reserve of energy for the next famine. The problem is there never is a famine. But your body doesn't know that. It is very obedient, and will do anything and everything to keep you alive. Whenever there is a surplus of food, it will get stored as fat for that day when there is no food.

Sugar in any form stimulates the release of insulin. Insulin is a hormone that is stored in your pancreas. Insulin then causes an enzyme by the name of lipoprotein lipase (LPL) to then store the excess sugar as fat.

Stress on the other hand stimulates the release of cortisol, which then stimulates LPL which, results in the storage of fat.

What constitutes stress in your body? Anything that elevates your cortisol. Things like caffeine, sleep deprivation, to much exercise, work stress, family stress, financial stress, marriage stress just to name a few. Yes , stress can make you fat. They key is to recognize it and work to minimize it.

The take home message is, in order to lose weight then we need to decrease our sugar intake and our stress.

Look for my graph and explanation on "Why and How the Body Stores Fat".
Awesome info with the FREE download on www.doctorisabel.com.

The Cheating Rule

We have to have a time when we can splurge. Like when you go out for a party or
you are at a nice restaurant with beautiful breads, desserts etc. For me it is usually on
a Friday evening when I have been good all week with my food intake, then I let it
go. I splurge and I do it without feeling guilty.

According to Dr. Heller at Mount Sinai Medical School in The Great Physician by
Jordan Rubin, we can eat whatever we want if it is done within one hour. The
rationale is this. They say since your body has been use to low levels of sugar then
less insulin is released therefore less fat is stored and more fat is used up for
immediate energy. However at 75 -90 minutes a second surge of insulin is released
which results in fat storage.

Bottom line: if you are going to indulge, you have one hour to do it. After one hour,
you will be packing it away as fat.

This does not imply to indulge everyday for one hour. This means if you need to go
for it, you can do it once in a while but just do it within an hour without feeling like
you blew it. As your health coach I also encourage you to be good to your body and
not pig out on fast food junk.

Ch 4. What Do I Eat Doc?

What is GI?

Every day your body has to take over 10,000 steps, think 40,000 thoughts,
pump 36,000 liters of blood round your system to keep you alive for the next
day. To do this it needs fuel and the fuel in the form of energy comes from
food.

Glucose is your body's preferred fuel source. It gets glucose from starches and sugars(carbohydrates) found in the food you eat every day. Glucose is made in the liver after your food has been digested in your stomach. The glucose is then sent to wherever it is needed in your body for energy. This energy could be use for running, thinking or it could be stored in muscles and fat for a later time.

The rate at which glucose goes into the bloodstream is called the the glycemic index.

• Low glycemic index (lo-GI foods) are converted slowly into glucose.

• Hi glycemic index (hi- GI foods) are converted quickly into glucose.

Insulin is a very important in this whole process. I consider insulin as the conductor of the orchestra. The glucose particles are the orchestra. When the glucose is released slowly (lo GI) there is no problem - the insulin has time to "think" about where that glucose is needed most and sends it there.

However, if high levels of glucose enter the bloodstream, the body panics. It might need some of the glucose for fuel, but to much can be harmful. The body therefore releases more insulin which quickly transfers the excess glucose to the fat stores where it can do no harm. As a result, we gain weight in the form of fat.

Weight gain isn't the only side effect of eating hi GI foods. If insulin levels are raised too often, then the cells that normally respond to glucose, laugh at the insulin and say " I am not paying attention to you anymore because you are always knocking on my door telling me to let the glucose in". Put another way, the cells become resistant to insulin's signals. This is called Insulin resistance.

Insulin resistance causes you to gain belly fat, raises your blood pressure, messes up your cholesterol, makes you infertile, kills your sex drive, makes you depressed, tired, demented and even causes cancer.

When glucose is not allowed into the cells then a problem arises. The glucose remains in the bloodstream and causes damage. Damage in the form of ageing and furring of the arteries. In addition, because the cells aren't getting enough fuel, which cause you to be tired, your body triggers the release of more and more insulin to try and fix up the problem. Over the years this triggers Type II Diabetes.

The goal is to switch to eating lo GI foods, which will cause a gentle rise of glucose in your bloodstream. This will result in a balanced system and weight loss.

Below is a list of foods grouped into the traffic light system.

• Lo GI foods are considered Green light : Eat as much as you want

• Medium GI foods are considered Yellow Light: Eat in moderation

• High GI foods are considered Red Light: Eat only as a treat

• Extra High GI foods are considered Flashing Red lights: Stay away

GI Food List

Lo GI / Green light: Eat large amounts

Vegetables ; Broccoli, asparagus, spinach, chard, kale, cabbage bokchoy, carrots, eggplant, cauliflower, mushrooms, capsicums, lettuce, green beans, onions, leeks, types of seaweed, celery, sprouts, artichoke, courgettes / zucchini, cucumber, endive,f ennel, garlic, leeks, rocket greens, watercress,r adicchio, radish, tomato, spinach, boiled sweet potato / kumara

Whole grains; oat bran, rolled oats, pearled barley, quinoa, buckwheat.

Legumes/ Nuts; Chickpeas, peanuts, walnuts, cashews, almonds, kidney beans, butter beans, navy beans, pinto beans, lentils, black beans, yellow spilt peas, soy beans

Fruit; Grapefruit, kiwi fruit, coconut, apple, avocado, all berries (like blueberries, strawberries, boysenberries, etc.), plum, green grapes, cherries

Protein; Please note that the folllowing are certainly categorized as lo-GI, however I caution you for the fat content. Anchovies, bacon, beef, chicken, clams, cod, crab, duck, eggs, gammon, haddock, halibut, ham, kippers, lamb, liver, lobster, mackerel, monkfish, mussels, pilchards, plaice, pork, prawns, salmon, sardines, sea bass skate, squid, sole, swordfish, trout, tuna, venison, veal.

Medium GI / Yellow light: Eat in moderation

Vegetables; Beets / Beetroot

Whole grains; Brown rice, basmati rice, black rice, red rice, couscous

Fruit; Peaches, nectarines, mango, apricots, pears, papaya, figs, melons, red grapes

High GI/ Red Light: eat only as a treat

Vegetables; baked potato, baked sweet potato /kumara , boiled potato , winter squash, peas, broad beans (fava) , pumpkin, turnips, yams

Whole grains; any rice that takes 10 minutes or less to cook, jasmine rice, sticky rice, millet

Fruit; Watermelon, dates, pineapple, bananas

*Did you know that one banana has 4.25 teaspoons of sugar?

Extra High GI / Flashing Red Light: stay away

Dried fruit and candy (lollies)

Drinks and GI

It is not just food that turns into glucose in your body, it is drinks too.

Below is a list from lo GI to high GI drinks.

Lo GI:

- Water
- Tea and herbal tea
- Milk
- Tomato juice
- Apple juice (without sugar)
- Carrot juice
- Pineapple juice (without sugar)
- Grapefruit juice (without sugar)
- Orange juice (without sugar)
- Cranberry juice (without sugar)
- Red wine
- White wine

- Cola

- Fizzy drinks

- High energy drinks

Hi GI:

• Beer

About Alcoholic drinks

Alcoholic drinks in the form of spirits such as gin, vodka and whiskey are also best avoided. While they have very little effect on insulin - they are technically low GI. However, the problem arises when one drinks, the appetite is increased which results in over eating. In addition high consumption of spirits is linked to other health problems.

Red wine is a better choice than spirits. Although it has a medium GI value, it contains antioxidants, which are good for your heart.

About fats

We need to also focus on which fats are safe to consume. There is a lot of confusion out there regarding what fats are ok to eat and which are ok to cook with. Below is a list for your kitchen.

Food Sources of GOOD and BAD Fats

GOOD Essential Fats;

Omega-3;

➢ *Flaxs*

- Soybean
- Walnuts
- canola organic expeller oil
- dark green leafy veggies
- cold water fish (cod, salmon, sardines, anchovies, tuna)
- pumpkin
- **Omega-6 :**
- Cold-pressed flax and sunflower oil
- cold-pressed high oleic safflower oil
- walnuts
- grapeseed oil
- sesame oil and tahini

GOOD Monounsaturated Fats:

- Extra-virgin cold-pressed olive oil
- sesame oil
- brazil nuts
- hazelnuts & filberts
- avocado
- peanuts and peanut butter (non-hydrogenated and no added sugar)
- cashews
- almond and almond butter
- macadamia nuts
- walnuts

- ➢ *pinon nuts*

- ➢ *soybean oil*

- ➢ *organic expeller-pressed canola oil*

GOOD Saturated Fats;

- > *Ghee (clarified butter)*

- ➢ *poultry (chicken and turkey)*

- > *coconut oil*

- ➢ *butter*

BAD Trans Fats; *Trans fats cause free radicals to be formed, which cause damage and aging of your body.*

> *Margarine*

> *hydrogenated peanut butter*

> *chocolate candy*

> *pastries & doughnuts*

> *commercially packaged cookies, crackers, and chips*

> *shortening*

> *any foods fried in shortening-type oils(deep-fried)*

> *Corn, sunflower, and canola oils that are not cold-pressed. (they contain hydrogenated or partially hydrogenated oils.*

BAD Saturated & Processed Fats;

- ➢ *shortening*

> all *"partially hydrogenated oils"*

> *rancid oils (exposed to oxygen, smell bad)*

   all oils left exposed to oxygen can go "rancid', which may be toxic to human tissue

> *poultry skin*

> *cheese*

> *red meats; beef, pork, lamb*

> *high temp deep-fried foods*

> *all "hydrogenated oils"*

Best oils to cook with at high temperature

>*Coconut oil*

>*Expeller or cold pressed Sesame Oil*

>*Expeller or cold pressed Sunflower Oil*

As you can see butter is better than margarine. Margarine is not a whole food, rather it is a trans fat which cause the formation of free radicals to form in your body which do all kinds of damage. Free radical formation, in particular causes your body to age in fast forward motion. If you put a block of margarine and butter out for the ants, they eat the butter and don't touch the margarine. So stay away from margarine and use butter.

But what about my cholesterol doc? Great question. There is recent research to indicate that we shouldn't be worried about our cholesterol as much as the things that cause inflammation. I will address inflammation in the next section. What is being found is half of all those who had a heart attack had normal cholesterol levels. So high cholesterol levels is NOT the cause of all the heart disease in the world.

5 messages to guide you to health

1. Raw is best. Try your hardest to eat foods in their natural state. Consider how old the food you are buying is. Typically it has taken at least one week to get to you so already, it's nutritional value has depleted by 40-50%. If you cook it, then again we have important enzymes and nutrients being destroyed.

If steaming a little is the best way to start your family on this journey, then I encourage that. We have a motto in our family to reach the goal and that goes like this "Whatever it takes". However the final goal is to eat foods in their freshest for, straight from the farmers field. If you can eat organic great. If not then you can do the following to clean your fruits and veggies:

• One part white vinegar to ten parts water. Let sit for few minutes then wash off.

This is the closest to getting the pesticides off our food.

2. Eat foods without labels or that don't come in a box, can or package. If they do have labels then you need to make sure to read the labels very carefully. Ideally you want less than 5 ingredients.

3. Stay away from the following ingredients.

• Foods with **preservatives, additives, coloring or dyes**. Anything you can't pronounce or recognize is a big no-no.

• Stay away from all foods that have **high fructose corn syrup**. Other disguised names for this are **corn syrup** or **sugar of maize** (maize is spanish for corn). This is an industrial food product, which is not natural. It is not a whole, real, fresh food and it lacks fiber or any nutritional value. In some cases there is mercury found as a by-product. Who needs it! If you want to avoid obesity, stay far away from it.

• All **white rice** and **white flour**. White rice and white flour stimulate insulin release and insulin's main purpose is to store fat for a future famine. It loves to store it where it can access it quickly like around the belly, upper arms, the back (lovingly called verandas).

• **Sugar** in the form of honey, agave, maple syrup, cane sugar or molasses. Sugar in any form also causes the rise on insulin, which causes the belly fat accumulation.

• Anything with "**Hydrogenated**" on it. This chemical process is just a way to add hydrogen atoms to fats so they can keep a longer shelf life. They have been known to cause heart disease and cancer. Most European countries and even

New York City have banned these fats and I encourage you to do the same for your health.

4. Fried foods and processed oils, such as corn, peanut, and canola. These are toxic fats when heated and full of free radicals, which can actually change good DNA into damaged DNA. There is no nutritional value in it so why even pour in into your tank?

5. Artificial Sweeteners such as

• Saccharin (sweet and low)

• anything that ends in "ol" like xylitol, sorbitol, mannitol, lactitol, and mailtol

• Acesulfame-k known as Ace-K, Sunette , Sweet and Safe (not!) and Sweet one. These all slow down your metabolism, make you hungry and make you fat. In one study, one group was given a diet drink everyday and the other group a non diet drink every day. At the end of the year, those who had the diet drink gained the most weight.

Ch 5 What is all this talk about inflammation?

As a medical doctor, I have been trained that a low fat and low cholesterol diet is the best prevention against heart disease, heart attacks, high blood pressure and obesity. After a patient was tested and found to have high cholesterol levels we then put them on a statin, which lowers the cholesterol levels and we started the patient on a low fat diet. Put so eloquently by Dr. Dwight Lundell, a heart surgeon in USA, "To deviate from this was considered heresy and could quite possibly result in malpractice."

The low fat low cholesterol plan is not working. Half of all those who have heart attacks have normal cholesterol levels. People are sicker now then ever before and what we now know is ,it is all preventable.

What do we know about the childhood problem? Childhood obesity has tripled from 1980 to 2010.

One on three children born today will have Type 2 Diabetes in their lifetime. Childhood obesity will have more impact on how long this generation will live than all other childhood cancers. Childhood Diabetes is a global problem.

60% of the worlds Type 2 Diabetics will be from Asia because it's the worlds largest region.

Fortunately there have been new studies, which show us that we had the low fat, low cholesterol plan ALL WRONG. Inflammation is the cause.

A mental picture of inflammation

Imagine a stiff brush rubbing on skin, over a short period of time. The skin breaks down and starts to bleed. This causes the body's repair system to come in and start repairing the area that was injured. During this time, he area becomes red, hot and swollen for a short period of time. This is the normal way our body repairs any injured site.

Now imagine this stiff brush rubbing on the skin over a long period of time. This time lets go to the inside of a blood vessel leading to your heart. What happens is the area becomes sticky and when cholesterol comes floating by it hooks on the sticky area on the blood vessel. After awhile more cholesterol hooks on and eventually blocks the blood vessel leading to the heart and then you get a heart attack. A heart attack is nothing more than a lack of blood supply to the heart muscle.

The main point here is this: **The cholesterol is not the problem, the stiff brush is.**

It is the stiff brush that started the whole problem. As for cholesterol, we need it for everyday life to make every living cell in our body. If I could take you and I into a living cell right now in your body, we would see that cholesterol makes the walls of the house. If we didn't have cholesterol, we couldn't be alive.

Who are the stiff brush players that are causing all this havoc in our body? Or put another way the contributors of Inflammation.

1. Sugar. Sugar is found in almost everything we eat. It is in bread, fast food with high fructose corn syrup, energy drinks, colas, pasta, and on and on and on. We know that sugar stimulates insulin, which does one of two things;

- It stores sugar into cells and when that is all done

- it stores sugar as fat. If you are insulin resistant than the sugar can't get into the cells and it stays in the blood stream.

   Sugar in the blood stream is dangerous because it starts scratching the inside line of the blood vessel. This is just like the stiff brush and makes it sticky and ready for cholesterol to hook on and cause problem.

   Sugar also wipes out your immune system for up to 2-4 hours after eating it. Your immune system is your army inside you, that attacks viruses and bacteria that come into your body. You don't want your army asleep when it's invaded by viruses and bacteria.

2. High fat foods. Especially trans- fats, saturated fats and processed fats like deep fried foods, we see and eat in fast food restaurants and take away fish and chip stores.

3. Food Allergens. People who are allergic to certain foods will have immune complexes form which lead to inflammation. Food allergens can be gluten, soy, dairy, peanut, eggs, and artificial sweeteners to name a few.

4. Insufficient fiber. Think of fiber as a broom in your gut that acts to sweep out toxins that cause inflammation.

5. Insufficient Phytonutrients. Phyto means plant. Phytonutrients are plant nutrients that are beneficial to you. Phytonutrients are found in fruits, vegetables, nuts and seeds that act to quench inflammation.

6. Insufficient exercise. Fat tissue helps to hide the contributors of inflammation. Exercising muscle reduces inflammation and improves insulin getting glucose into cells.

7. Vitamin D3 deficiency. This important vitamin has been found to be a prime player in the prevention of inflammation. More on this in detail in Part 7; Chapter 2.

8. Emotional Stress. Emotional stress and toxic relationships promote inflammation, slows down wound healing and cause your immune system to be suppressed.

The bottom line is that it is not the fat or the cholesterol in our diets that is causing Heart Disease, High Blood Pressure, Type 2 Diabetes, Strokes, Obesity and Alzheimer's Disease. The real cause is inflammation. People have been on a low fat low cholesterol diet for 6 decades and it just is not working.

What do we do? Eat foods that your great- great grandmother would recognize.

Part 2: Healthy Shopping <><><><>

Chapter1. What to Have in Your Kitchen

It's time to get your kitchen ready for your success. I suggest getting rid of all the bad stuff and investing in all the good stuff for your health and future. You are worth it.

Utensils:

• Blender

• Non Aluminum cooking pans

• Wooden cutting board

• Sharp knives

• Measuring spoons

Spices: Make sure these don't have any preservatives or sugar added to them

• Salt

• Pepper

• Oregano

• Basil

• Paprika

• Cumin

• Paprika

• Chili Powder

• Curry Powder

• Rosemary

• Cinnamon

• Turmeric

Oils/Sauces to have on hand:

• Extra Virgin Olive Oil cold pressed

• Organic Soy or Tamari sauce (wheat free)

• Coconut Oil

• Sesame Oil Cold pressed

• Sunflower oil Cold pressed

• Balsamic vinegar

• Butter

Pantry:

- Garlic Cloves

- Sweet potatoes/Kumara

- Red and White onions

- Ginger root

Tea:

- Organic Green Tea

- Peppermint tea

- Ginger tea

Nuts: Raw not roasted as roasted cuts down on nutritional value.

- Almonds

- Walnuts

- Brazil Nuts

- Peanuts (if not allergic)

- Pine nuts

- Chia Seeds

- Sesame seeds

- Sunflower seeds

- Pumpkin seeds

- Macadamia nuts

- Coconut (shredded , without sugar)

- Pecans

Grains:

- Brown rice
- Red Rice
- Black Rice
- Quinoa
- Oats

Legumes/Beans: (Canned is ok)

- Chickpeas
- Kidney beans
- Black beans
- Butter beans
- Lentils
- Navy Beans
- Pinto Beans
- Yellow split beans
- Soy beans

Misc:

- Coconut milk (without sugar)
- Almond milk (without sugar)
- Hemp milk
- Oat milk
- Tahini (ground sesame)
- Organic Almond butter

- Organic Peanut butter

- Anchovy

- Capers

- Mustard

- Mayonnaise (without sugar)

- Tomato sauce

Breakfast Cereal:

Have a rolled oat cereal on hand without sugar for kids.

Refrigerator:

- Grapefruit

- Kiwi fruit

- Strawberries

- Blueberries

- Boysenberry

- Grapes

- Apple

- Cherries

- Peaches

- Nectarines

- Mango

- Apricots

- Pears

- Papaya

- Melon
- Broccoli
- Asparagus
- Spinach
- Chard
- Kale
- Cabbage
- Bok Choy
- Carrots
- Eggplant
- Cauliflower
- Mushrooms
- Red Pepper/ Capsicums
- Lettuce
- Green beans
- Leeks
- Celery
- Sprouts
- Artichoke
- Courgettes/Zucchini
- Cucumber
- Endive
- Fennel
- Rocket greens
- Watercress

- Radicchio

- Radish

- Beets/ Beetroot

- Celery

Protein:

- Eggs

- Chicken breasts

- Tofu

- Salmon

- Tuna

- Clams

- Mussels

- Fish

- Grass fed Beef

- Lamb

- Duck

Chapter 2. Places Where Sugar Hides

I met up with one of my clients for health coaching I asked her to remove sugar from her life. She so innocently said to me, " Oh I never add sugar to anything." I lovingly looked at her and said, "You don't have to, the food industry does it for you.".

It is almost a requirement to have a Phd. to go shopping nowadays with all the different aliases that sugar has. Below is a list for you to have while you go shopping. Even my 13 year old patients carry it with them, and are so excited being on the hunt for sugar in their food, because they know that sugar stimulates insulin release, which causes more belly fat to be stored.

Places where sugar hides:

- Agave syrup or Agave sugar (yes, agave has a low GI, however what it dies it far worse than raise insulin levels. It also increases your triglyceride levels which trigger inflammation and damage your liver)

- Barley malt

- Beet sugar

- Brown sugar

- Buttered syrup

- Cane juice crystals

- Cane sugar

- Caramel

- Corn syrup

- Corn syrup solids

- Confectioner's sugar

- Carob syrup

- Castor sugar

- Date sugar

- Demerara sugar

- Dextran

- Dextrose

- Diastatic malt

- Diatese

- Dried fruit (hi glucose and is concentrated sugar)

- Ethyl maltol
- Fructose
- Fruit Juice
- Fruit juice concentrate
- Galactose
- Glucose
- Glucose solids
- Golden sugar
- Golden syrup
- Grape sugar
- High fructose corn syrup (HFCS)
- Sugar of maize
- Honey
- Icing sugar
- Invert sugar
- Lactose
- Maltodextrin
- Maltose
- Malt syrup
- Maple syrup
- Molasses
- Muscovado sugar
- Panocha
- Raw sugar
- Refiner's syrup

- Rice syrup

- Sorbitol

- Sorghum syrup

- Sucrose

- Sugar

- Treacle

- Turbinado sugar

- Xylitol

- Yellow sugar

- Anything ending in "ose" is a sugar

Now the question arises," what can I use as a sweetener"? I always recommend **Stevia**. Stevia a plant from the sunflower family and is 300 times sweeter than sugar. It is low GI and if you need something as a sweetener, then Stevia is your best option. This is what we use in our family. I prefer the drops as I can control the sweetness more readily.

Chapter 3, What Foods to Buy

Making the decision to take better care of yourself, through healthy eating is the first step. I always like to think of my body as a car, if I pour concrete into the gasoline tank, I won't get very far. However, when I "fill her up" with high octane, I will get far. The same philosophy applies to our body.

I was born in 1959, and I am just about to turn 53 years young. My family is from Cuba, and in Cuba the cars last a long time. If I were to consider myself like a 1959 Ford Fairlane, and I had to make it last for a long time, then I would take really good care of myself.

I haven't always filled my tank with high octane. I wasn't even in the right head-space to do that, especially during my medical education. Breakfast for me was dessert; a strong cup of coffee and a muffin. We know, that my blood sugars after that nutritious breakfast were falling after 1.5 hour. Nothing a handful of skittles, and another cup of coffee couldn't handle, which would hold me over for another 1.5 hours.

Roller coaster blood sugars not only feel bad, they just play havoc with your emotions. Think about our kids who are in school, who have had dessert for breakfast. I use to see out my window, kids going to school with bags of chips, and an energy drink. Not only would I feel sorry for the kids, but also for the poor teachers. It is impossible for the kids to concentrate. Hence the reason to recreate your new health strategy, and reposition yourself for better health.

Repositioning yourself and your family is a little tricky. It is much like taking a ocean liner ship, and making a 180 degree turn. A maneuver like that does not occur quickly. I remember when I foolishly announced to my teenage daughters that I was not going to buy anymore sugar. I was crucified! It was like taking away a drug from the drug addict. And in a way, I was.

Like Robert Kiyosaki says, "You either win or you learn". I learned that I shouldn't have announced my new commitment to the Hunsinger Home of "no sugar".....I should have just quietly implemented it. Allow yourself time for the re-position. Once completed, you will be on the right track.

In regards to buying organic.

I am completely amazed at how expensive organic food can be at times. I would purposely avoid going into the organic shops because I thought it was only for the rich who could afford to waste their money on expensive foods. Remember, I did my pre-med degree in Boulder, Colorado.

However after reading and researching I have learned so much more about organic food. The organic farmer is held to another set of stringent rules, and are not subsidized by the government. In addition, they produce a higher quality of food, that does not have chemicals, nor is it genetically modified (GMO). Quite honestly, I cannot unlearn what I have learned. I would be lying to you if I coached you otherwise. When possible, I would encourage you to buy organic. You are worth the investment. If it is difficult to purchase organic greens and vegetables, as it occurs with us, then you can clean them with one part white vinegar and 10 parts water. Just swish around for a few minutes then rinse in water. That process will help remove most of the pesticides. Remember, we do whatever we have to, to achieve the goal. Step by step.

Part 3: Healthy Cooking with Chef Michael

Yummy food that your body and family will love. ◇◇◇

Chapter 1. Kitchen Essentials and Time-Saving Tips

Here is a list of my kitchen essentials:

• Sharp set of knives

• cutting board (preferably 2; one for protein, one for all the rest)

• Food processor

• drink blender

• utensils: whisk, spoon, spatula, etc.

• fresh herbs and spices, including sea salt and black pepper

• fresh garlic and ginger

• set of bowls for mixing

• set of measuring cups and spoons

• extra virgin olive oil (cold pressed) for non-cooking recipes

• sesame oil and coconut oil for cooking

Time Saving Tips for a Busy Life

It seems with all the wonderful gadgets and modern conveniences, that life should be simpler and full of free time. However I've noticed that most people are busier today than life was 20 years ago. One of the pleasures of our day that is getting missed is "eating Healthy Real Food Meals" during our day. I'm not going to try and analyze why this is happening (I do have my opinion on this). Let's look at some techniques that will help you organize your time in the kitchen, so hopefully you can sit, relax, and enjoy Real 100% Food.

• prepare a mixed raw vegetable platter on Sunday and Thursday with a dipping sauce or hummus. This will allow the family to have a healthy snack ready at all times to be eaten at home or taken to school or work. (prep time, about 1 hour); tomato quarters, carrot and celery sticks, broccoli and cauliflower lightly steamed and cooled, capsicum strips(bell pepper), zucchini strips(courgette),etc...

• soups, sauces, and salads; I like to prepare these items in larger quantities to last a few days. Soups and sauces can be frozen and used another time. Salads are great for 2 days without the lettuce (which will wilt)

• prepare a few extra portions when making a main type of dish and freeze some. Generally, if I'm going to take the time to cook and get into the kitchen, then I want to make my time count. It doesn't take more time to prepare extra when I already have the ingredients and food cooking. It's pretty much same time to make 2 liters of soup, as to make 1 liter of soup.

Chapter 2. Breakfast, Important Start for your Day

Breakfast is the most important meal of the day, it jump starts your metabolism and gets bodily functions on the correct path for the day. Start you day with a healthy breakfast within 1 hour of awakening, and you will have an energized, healthy, tuned-in day. Here are some guidelines to start your day:

Breakfast Recipes/Ideas:

Protein Shake: we recommend using a dairy free or whey protein.

Healthy Starter:

• 1-2 scoops protein powder

• mixed fruit berries, 2 cup

• tahini paste, 1 Tbs.

• chia seeds, 2 Tbs. (high in omega-3 fatty acids and fiber)

- pinch of cinnamon

- non-dairy milk 2 cups (almond, rice, coconut, hemp > all without sugar)

- water or ice cubes 2 cups

- Blend all in drink mixer and enjoy. Makes 2 -3 servings

Mocha-Blueberry:

- 1-2 scoops of protein powder

- 1 cup of blueberries

- 1 cup organic decaf plunger or espresso coffee

- pinch of cinnamon

- 2 Tbs. chia seeds

- 2 cups non dairy milk

- 2 cups water or ice

- blend all, and makes 2-3 servings

Strawberry-Coconut Desire:

- Use the healthy starter recipe with these changes:

- only strawberries for fruit

- use coconut milk

- add 2tbs of coconut flakes

- blend all, and makes 2-3 servings

Vegetable Frittata: (no crust quiche), can be made the day before and reheated

Ingredients:

- 10 eggs whisked in bowl

- 2 cups diced vegetables

- 2 garlic cloves chopped

- 2 Tbs. fresh chopped parsley

- 2 Tbs. fresh chopped basil

- 1 Tbs. dry dill leaf

- salt and pepper to taste

How to:

- Saute veggies for 3 minutes with garlic and herbs. When done, combine veggie and egg mixture in a lightly buttered baking pan. bake in oven at 150*C (325*F) for 25-35 min. (Nice golden brown)

Suggested Flavors: bacon or ham, grated cheese, salmon pieces, mushrooms, capsicum, onion, courgettes, tomato.

Plain Greek Yogurt:

Another great option for breakfast is plain Greek yoghurt. Greek yoghurt has more protein then regular yoghurt, and by adding a few ingredients you can have a protein filled meal. Add flaxseed or chia seeds for the omega-3's, fresh berries, organic muesli mix, and 2 drops Stevia for sweetness.

Quick and Easy: if you want to keep it simple; have two eggs poached on 1 piece of gluten free buttered toast. That will do you for the morning.

Part 3: chapter 3. Juice Recipes for Fast/Cleanse

In 2012, Michael and I, along with some friends from around the world, did a 10-day juice fast. Yes, no chewing of food for 10 days, yes, just real 100% juice. Before you turn off thinking,"that is crazy", please understand this type of decision is only done with a true beneficial reason. The health reasons for a juice fast are many, and your body will truly love what it does for your organs. If you want to have a fun read about the 10-day fast; we did daily posts on our blog at www.doctorisabel.com. You can search for 10-day fast, or go back to August 2012, and you can follow the process. We have decided to keep our Tuesdays as Juice fast day, as we love the cleansing, and energizing effect we get during this process. Here are some recipes we have used for our juice fast. I hope you enjoy them if you choose to Juice:

Quick tips;

- When the recipe calls for fruit, please have fruit be maximum of 20% of blend.

- Using wheatgrass gives a High octane of nutrients to any Juice.

- Adding cracked black pepper and sea salt adds to the flavor

Juices:

- The Kiwiana: Blend of beetroot (red beets), kale, red radishes, carrots, and apples

- Morning Zinger: Apples, carrots, celery, orange, fresh ginger

- The Thirst Quencher: green apple, kale or spinach, cucumber, celery, lime

- The italian: tomatoes, capsicum (bell pepper), spinach or kale, celery, garlic clove, fresh basil, fresh parsley,

- The Latin Fire: tomatoes, cucumber, spinach or kale, celery, carrots, fresh chili peppers, garlic clove, pinch of cumin seed, pinch of smoked paprika

Part 3: Chapter 4. Soups, Sauces, Dips

Let's have fun with soups, sauces, and dips. This is one of my favorite areas of food, because we can experiment with so may flavors. All of the recipes can be made in bulk, so you can freeze them for future use. I will add some flavor suggestions to each recipe, however please feel free to try new tastes on your own.

Sauces & Dips:

Traditional Hummus:

This is one of my favorite foods, because it has the combination of protein, carbs, and good fats. Can be used as a spread for sandwiches, or as a dip for veggies and crackers.

Ingredients:

2 cups cooked or canned garbanzo beans, ½ cup liquid from beans,

Juice of 1 lemon, 1 clove garlic, 2tbs. chopped parsley, 2 tbs. extra virgin olive oil,

2 tbs. tahini, salt and pepper to taste.

How to: puree all ingredients in food processor

Suggested Flavors: sundried tomatoes, roasted red capsicum, diced beetroot, rocket leaves, olives, extra garlic clove.

Basic Aioli:

Ingredients: 4 egg yolks, 2 cups extra virgin olive oil, 1 garlic clove, juice of 1 lemon, salt & pepper to taste.

How to: puree all ingredients except oil in food processor, then slowly add oil to puree until desired thickness. (listen to machine start to work harder as the aioli thickens)

Suggested Flavors: capsicum or chilies, olives, fresh basil or parsley, extra garlic clove, fresh coriander, fresh lime juice.

Traditional Pasta/ Pizza sauce:

Ingredients for 8 servings;

1 diced onion, 4 garlic cloves, about 12 fresh basil leaves chopped, small bunch fresh parsley chopped, 6 large diced tomatoes or 2 cans of chopped tomatoes, salt and pepper to taste.

How To:

Saute all ingredients except tomatoes for 3-5 minutes, add tomatoes, turn down low, and let simmer for 30 minutes.

Suggested Flavors:

fresh oregano, fresh thyme, different types of tomatoes, add some chopped courgette (zucchini), or diced carrots and capsicum (bell peppers).

Soups: Soup is another one of my favorites. I will give a basic recipe to start with, and then you can have fun from there. Soups are inexpensive ways to feed the family healthy in all times of the year. Just use the products that are in season.

Quick/Simple vegetable Soup:

Ingredients; About a litre or medium bowl of coarsely chopped vegetables, a litre of vegetable stock, herbs and spices to taste.

How To; Sauté vegetables, herbs, and spices in large pot for about 5 minutes. Add stock and simmer for 30 minutes. Puree in drink blender or food blending hand held stick to desired thickness. Season to taste to finish.

Hot Tip; Add kumara (yams) or cauliflower to vegetable mix, as they are slightly starchy and will thicken the soup naturally. Have fun and use many types and flavors of vegetables and fresh herbs.

Asian Tum-Yum soup:

Ingredients for 2 liters:

2 cups thinly sliced or diced chicken, 1-2 chopped hot chili (depending on your heat taste level), julienne of 1 red and 1 green capsicum, 1 carrot diced or asian cut, 2 sticks celery asian cut or diced, 1 cup sliced shitake mushrooms, 1/4 cup green peas, 1/4 cup sliced green onions, 1 liter chicken stock, 2 cans coconut creme, 4tbs fresh grated ginger, 6 cloves garlic, salt and pepper to taste.

How To: Saute chicken, vegetables and spices for 5 minutes, add stock, continue to let soup simmer for 15 minutes, then add coconut crème and lime juice, season to taste, simmer for 15-30 minutes more. You can take 25% of soup and blend in drink blender. Add the mix back into the soup to thicken, and finish.

Chapter 5. Lunch/Dinner

Yes, I have put lunch and dinner sections together, with a purpose. In the western diet, we seem to pack in most of our food intake at the end of our waking day. This isn't the healthy way to distribute our daily calorie intake. And many people through more down just before going to bed. This is like throwing a huge log on a fire with low embers. You loose the fire and just get smoke.

For us, that means we are storing fat at the end of the day, because we aren't moving much (usually sitting watching TV). Unless you are doing a Tango competition from 9pm-midnight, you won't be burning much energy after 8pm. We should have about 70% of our daily calorie intake by the time we have our dinner. So let's look at the lunch/dinner recipes as interchangeable.

Stir-fry Chicken:

Ingredients;

• Marinated Chicken pieces (marinate in coriander, lime, garlic, coconut cream or coconut milk, fresh ginger, tamari or soy sauce)

• mixture of sliced and diced veggies

• brown, log-grain, red, or black rice.

How to: stir-fry chicken in hot pan using coconut, sesame, or sunflower oil for 2-3 minutes, then add mixture of raw veggies. Stir-fry hot for about 5 minutes, (try not to overcook the mix). Serve with cooked rice.

Suggested Flavors: celery, carrot, capsicum, green beans, broccoli, mushrooms, courgette, leeks, red onion, chili peppers. Have fun with your veggie mix, by using different types of cuts.

Greek Salad:

Ingredients;

• 1 red onion,

• 1 red capsicum,

• 1 green capsicum,

• 2 tomatoes,

• 1 cucumber (all coarsely chopped)

• handful of pitted green and black olives

• 50grams of feta cheese.

For salad dressing: juice of 1 lemon, 1 crushed garlic clove, 1tbs. oregano, 1tbs. chopped parsley, 1/4 cup extra virgin olive oil, cracked black pepper and sea salt to taste.

How to; in small mixing bowl, mix all salad dressing ingredients except oil. Then using a whisk, slowly blend in olive oil. In large salad bowl mix vegetables, herbs, spices, and olives. Pour salad dressing over vegetable mix to desired wetness.

Suggested Serving; Place Cos (romaine) lettuce leaves around edge of serving platter, place salad mix in middle, and top with crumbled feta cheese and chopped parsley leaves.

Quinoa Salad w/avocado & black beans:

Ingredients:

• 1 cup quinoa

• 1 1/2 c. water

• 1 chopped scallion (green onion)

- 1/2 diced red capsicum (bell pepper)

- 1 sliced tomato

- 1 sliced avocado

- 1 cup black beans (cooked)

- 2 limes

- fresh cilantro

- olive oil to taste

- fresh rocket or spinach greens

How To:

Cook quinoa in lightly simmering water (salt and pepper to taste) for 5 minutes. Turn off heat and allow to sit ,covered for about 10-12 more minutes until water is absorbed. Some veggie stock or some butter in water for flavor is nice.

When quinoa is cool, combine with juice of 1 lime, red capsicum, scallion, 2 Tbs. olive oil, 1 Tbs. chopped cilantro, pinch of dried cumin. Toss all ingredients in bowl.

To Serve:

On serving tray place greens around edge, then alternate tomato and avocado slices to from colorful pattern. Place quinoa mixture in middle of platter, sprinkle black beans around edges and garnish with sprinkle of chopped cilantro and lime wedges. Drizzle some olive oil on greens and tomato/avocado pattern.

Coleslaw:

Ingredients:

- 1/2 head green cabbage shredded

- 1/4 head red cabbage shredded

- 2 carrots shredded

- 1 red onion diced small

- 1 green capsicum diced small

- 1 /2 cup basic aioli

- juice of 1 lemon

- fresh dill, parsley, salt, pepper to taste

Combine all ingredients in mixing bowl, and serve as side dish with main course. Makes enough for about 10 servings

Baked Fresh Salmon Filet:

The salmon can be eaten warm after baking, or cooled and eaten for salads, or with eggs for breakfast. Great protein dish full of Omega 3 fatty acids. I like to cook a large piece to have for meals over a day or two.

Ingredients:

- whole boneless salmon side/skin on

- 1 lemon

- fresh or dry dill weed

- smoked paprika

How to:

Lightly grease baking pan with sesame or coconut oil. Place salmon filet on pan, spread spices, herbs, salt and pepper, and juice of lemon over salmon. Bake in oven @ 150*C for about 15-20 minutes. The meat will be a lovely pink color when finished. When cooled, the meat will come off the skin easily if desired.

Fish and Chips:

Yes, I know, how can that be healthy? Well, here is an alternative that is tasty, and remains nutritious.

Ingredients:

- 4 pieces firm white flesh fish of your choice

- 3 golden kumara (yams) cut in wedges

- gluten free flour

- gluten free bread crumbs

- 2 eggs for egg-wash

- sesame or coconut oil

How to:

Dredge fish in flour, then into egg-wash (mixture of eggs and water), then into bread crumbs. Place on plate and chill for 1 hour to set.

Cut kumara into wedges, about 1/8 the size. Toss them in a mix of paprika, garlic, chili powder, salt, and pepper, and 1Tbs. sesame oil.

Bake kumara in 180*C oven for about 20 minutes

Fry the fish filets in sesame or coconut oil for 5 minutes, until golden brown.

Serve with aioli, or a wasabi-mayo, and of course if you like Ketchup.

Chicken Caesar Salad:

This is a classic salad that can be a main meal for lunch or dinner. You might also omit the chicken, and use as a side salad for the main meal. You could substitute salmon for chicken for a twist.

Ingredients:

- 2 cups of diced or julienned chicken meat

- 2 pieces of gluten free bread

- fresh parmesan cheese

- 4 whole eggs

- caesar-style aioli

- 1 head cos lettuce (romaine)

How To:

Wash, clean, and chop lettuce coarsely. Drain off excess water, and set aside.

For the Caesar dressing; Use basic aioli recipe, with addition of anchovy filets, 1 extra garlic clove, and some parmesan cheese.

Cut the bread into cubes and toss with enough melted butter to lightly moisten. Saute in pan until nice golden brown for croutons. Cook the chicken meat and set aside. Poach the eggs and set aside.

To Serve:

Toss lettuce leaves, chicken, and croutons in mixing bowl with enough aioli to flavor them. Place mix on platter, place 1 poached egg on top per serving, and sprinkle grated parmesan over top. Serves 4 side salads or 2 main meals.

Part 4: Why Winners Win

The Mental Game of Winning Health <><><><>

Chapter1 Attitude

The problem is not the problem. The problem is your attitude about the problem.

Do you understand?"

-Captain Jack Sparrow

Why do some people win and some people lose? I believe it all has to do with the person's attitude.

Here is a true life example that I just experienced the other day while Michael and I were out on a walk. It was a beautiful warm sunny spring Saturday afternoon. I was in the middle of writing this book and Michael had a lot of projects on the go. Michael is a peaceful, pleasant, easy-going and adaptable person. He also is fun, outgoing and optimistic. Nothing much rocks his boat. I to am fun, outgoing, and optimistic, however my stronger personality trait of being goal-oriented and bossy has a tendency of taking over me. And so it did on this walk. In the middle of the walk I said, "OK, when we get back, we are going to buckle down and get to work." Michael smiled and said, "I prefer to say, I am going to enjoy the day." I was thinking about getting serious and buckling down and getting some work done. Someone once said, writing books is like having homework the rest of your life. I can truly relate to this. And so, this attitude brought on a surge of anxiety in my heart. Michael's attitude, on the other hand, still wanted to reach his goal of getting work done, but it was by enjoying the journey. I thank God for bringing a man into my life that brings peace and helps me think about what I am thinking about.

Bottom line is attitude is the mental gymnastics we play. It is our thought life turned inside out. So depending on how you think will determine how you live your life. Either enjoying the journey, or dreading it. Most people's minds are like a wild untamed animal. You just have to learn to tame your mind. You have to crave and pursue the taming of your mind. That is work because it is an everyday event. Trust me, I constantly have to think about what I am thinking. If my mind is not on the right track to reach my goal, then I have change what I am saying to myself.

We have control of two things in this world; our thoughts and our attitude. Those two determine where we go and where we end up.

I am always amazed and excited when I meet, or read of someone who had terrible circumstances, but decided to take control of their thoughts and attitude and become an over comer.

Chris Gardner is a perfect example. He is portrayed in the movie, In pursuit of happyness. He was a hard working man, but due to circumstances, found himself homeless with his two year old son. He could have very easily played the victim, however he made the choice to not play that card. Instead he made the choice to fight for his son's, and his life, and now he is a very successful entrepreneur, investor, and international inspirational speaker.

Do you know when someone says, " That person has a good attitude?" That statement means they are positive, delightful, and you want to be around them. When they pass you buy, they leave a beautiful smelling perfume in their trail. On the other hand, when someone says, "That person has a bad attitude?", that entails they are negative, nasty, and you just don't want to be around them. Everything is a drama or nightmare when they are around. When they pass you by, their perfume is simply and quite honestly; nauseating and revolting. We all have people like that in our lives. Where does that come from? It comes from the choices they make.

It is our responsibility to take control of our thoughts and attitude. We have the control, no one else. Next we are going to see how we can tame our thoughts to cause us to win. Win with our health, win with our relationships, win in life.

Part 4. Chapter 2. Your Thinking Mind and Your Thinking Heart.

If you think right, you work right."

- Dr. Amen

Why is it that some people can lose weight and keep it off, while others lose the weight and it eventually comes back? It all has to do with our thinking.

A story that comes to mind was one of the contestants in the Biggest Loser. He went into the competition with the goal in mind to win the whole thing. He lost 174 lbs (79 kg), but he didn't win the competition and felt like a failure. Six months later , he regained 116 lbs (53 kgs). Why? Because no one taught him how to think. Truly, if you think right, you work right.

How do we think right?

I want you to imagine a big balloon. Now imagine two big balloons. One represents your head, and the other your heart. Got it? Next make a horizontal line across both balloons. The top part is your conscious (the part of your you that you are aware of) and below the line is your unconscious, (the part of you that you are not aware of like your breathing, heart rate and your temperature). The brain balloon, we will call Your thinking mind. The heart balloon, we will call Your thinking heart. Stay with me, we need to get the basics down before we go on with this analogy, even If you have to draw a picture of a head and a heart. The line that goes across the middle of your brain and heart we will call a door. And this door is always open. Whatever the top part of your brain and heart hear will also be placed in the bottom part.

Remember the door that connects the top to the bottom part of your brain and heart is always open and both are thinking...the thinking brain and the thinking heart. Now let's drop a thought into your brain and heart. Consider the thought, a seed. All seeds (thoughts) get planted in the conscious part and over time take root in the subconscious part. Since the door is always open, then we can say that all thoughts will take root over time in the subconscious.

The soil in the subconscious of your brain and your heart is very obedient, and will grow anything you plant. If you plant a corn seed, you will get a corn plant. Equally if you plant a hemlock seed, which by the way is a poison, and can kill people, then it will grow a hemlock plant. The subconscious ground cannot tell the difference between a "good for you seed" like corn; versus a "not so good for you seed."

The same principle applies to our thoughts. Every thought is like a seed, and it will bear certain fruit. It can bring about a positive result or a negative result. It is your choice.

Every decision has a future attached to it. Every seed you allow to take root will bear fruit. Good seeds have good futures attached to it. Bad seeds have a bad future attached to it.

What are you planting?

Have you ever heard the saying "what you think about, comes about?" This is so true. You can always tell what people are thinking about and/or feeling because of what comes out of their mouth.

• If a person chooses to plant jealous seed then they talk envy.

• If a person chooses to plant a grateful seed then they talk joy.

• If a person chooses to plant the "I can do it !!!" seed then they talk about overcoming and winning.

Your chances of success are actually based on what you say to yourself. A study done to show the percentage of success on what people would say when asked if they would succeed proved this.

• "I won't" resulted in 0% success

• "I can't" .... 10% success

• "I don't know how".. 20%

- "I wish I could" 30%

- "I want to"..............40%

- "I think I might".......50%

- "I might".................60%

- "I think I can"..........70%

- "I can"....................80%

- "I am" 90%

- "I did".....................100%

The key is to plant seeds that are in the "I am" category claiming who the new recreated and reposition you is. Thought like I am a winner, I am diligent, I am healthy. Do your best to reject thoughts of limitation and failure in your mind and heart, and replace them with words of victory, health, success, and joy.

Making sure your mind and heart are in sync.

It is important to realize that your mind and your heart are a mastermind team. A mastermind is a collection of harmonious co-operation of two or more, who ally themselves for the purpose of accomplishing any given task. In the business world like Apple, they have a mastermind team to create a successful product. It is important to have all members on the mastermind team on the same page instead of sabotaging each other. For instance, in your head you can say "I am going to lose weight" but your heart's thoughts are "It will never happen." Well guess what, the negative wins.

Another example is my daughter who was learning how to drive a manual (stick shift) car at 16 years. She would tell herself she could do it, but hear heart thought differently and she would tell herself "I can't, I am afraid" and she froze. After a little love and encouragement, she was able to get her mind and heart mastermind heading in the right direction and she passed her test and got her learner's license.

Getting the heart and mind to move in unison toward your goal is paramount to your success in whatever you do. My recommendation, is to listen to what you are thinking about, and listen to what you are saying. If they are mirroring each other, then all is good. But if they aren't, then you need to work on either your heart or your mind.

Chapter 3. Forgiveness as a Cure

Imagine someone does something to you and hurts your feelings. For instance, they said something insensitive to you. Or say someone promised you something, and they didn't live up to the promise. Now, every time you see them your stomach churns, the hairs on your neck stand up, and you wish nothing but doom and gloom to happen to them.

Guess what? You have just allowed the seed of unforgiveness to take root into your subconscious soil.

What fruit is produced when we plant this seed?

• unhappiness

• anger

• victim mentality

• depression

• bitterness

• guilt

• bondage

• suppressed immune system

• frown wrinkles on our face

Realistically, when we are full of unforgiveness it is like us drinking poison and expecting it will harm the other person. We need to do ourselves a favor, and save a lot of time and anger by forgiving. How do you know when you need to forgive someone more? Very easy, when you see, think, or hear that person, and you feel anger, rage or hate, then you need to keep on forgiving.

I realize that humans do some terrible things. I am not making light of your hurts that have occurred to you. I too have planted many seeds of unforgiveness. However when I realized how it hurts me more than it hurts the other person, I soon realized it was a losing investment. The problem with people is, they are "so people", and they don't think about what their words or actions do to us. Still to this day, I have to be very aware to not allow the seed of unforgiveness to take root and grow its huge tree in my heart. The good news is, "We are in control now!" and we know the signs. We can pull this out by the roots, either when it is a small seedling, or when it is an enormous tree, with a well entrenched root system. It's our choice.

My recommendation to you is keep on forgiving until you don't have to forgive any more. You will know this when you see, think, or hear the person that offended you, and you feel love and peace. Yes, it may take some time but keep at it...this too is good for your healing. I call it your emotional health.

"Listen carefully, you need to forgive to free your own life up. When you forgive someone, you are exhibiting the most God like character and with it comes a peace that surpasses no understanding. Trust me , I have had to do a lot of it."

- **John Maxwell, worldwide leadership authority**

Chapter 4   What to Say

Did you know that your life is like a blank canvas and you have the paint brush? What kind of life are you painting? I hope to coach you to paint a healthy life. Painters see it on the inside before they actually paint the picture. Here is a story, which shows this powerful principle.

There was this woman who lost 100 lbs (45 kg). She was beautiful, happy and now very confident. When asked how she did it she said, " I tried diet after diet without results. The key was not to diet, but to see myself at a certain weight first." She saw herself at a particular weight in her mind's canvas, which was then painted onto her life canvas.

That brings me to my next question. What are you seeing on the inside? Are you seeing breast cancer, diabetes, even a heart attack? Are you saying I will never get rid of this weight? I will always be a smoker. You don't have to be sick! 80% of chronic disease is preventable through lifestyle changes.

You don't have to have diabetes type 2, high blood pressure, high cholesterol, cancer, and even Alzheimer's disease. Did you know that. I honestly didn't until I became a member of The Institute of Functional Medicine. It was there that I have been exposed to getting to the root cause of disease. And that is why I am here now to bring you hope for a healthier future.

After I finished my medical training and practiced medicine for 10 or so years, I just thought we give people pills to cure them. It was a revelation when I realized we don't have a healthcare system, we have disease management and I was one of those managers. I hated it. I became a doctor to help people be their best, not manage their dis-ease.

I would like to share with you what I am saying to myself everyday with translates into the picture I paint for my life. The goal is to give you an idea of the sorts of statement you can say to yourself also known as positive affirmation. Because what we think about, comes about:

• I am strong, toned and full of energy.

• I am getting prettier and prettier everyday.

• I am safe for success.

• I am healthy.

Do you get the idea? Do you see what you can be or do you see what you can't be? You are the painter with the brush and canvas right in front of you.

Below are a few affirmations you might wish to use or add to. The purpose is to give you ideas from which you can create your own unique affirmations. That's how I did it. I built my own on the words from others.

Remember: If you can change your words, you can change your world.

Here goes;

- I am making a positive difference in people's lives.

- I am clear about my goals but I am flexible about how I achieve it.

- I believe.

- I am like a tree in the wind, I bend but I don't break.

- Success does not happen by accident.

- I am positive.

- I can do this. (and I have a set of stairs going up next to the statement for a visual affect)

- Winners never quit and quitters never win.

- I am a winner.

- I become what I think about.

- My prosperity is good for all people.

- "When I have finally decided that a result is worth getting. I go ahead on it and make trial after trial until it comes." Thomas Edison

- Whatever I passionately pursue, I will possess.

- My playing small serves no one.

- Everyday and in every way I am becoming better and better.

- I don't have to believe every stupid thought that I think.

- I am an over comer.

- Don't break ...bounce.

- I love public speaking.

- I add value to people's lives.

The list can go on and on and on and,............. well you know what I mean.

The bottom line, my friend, is this,

"Be careful how you are talking to yourself, because you are listening'

-Lisa M. Hayes

I encourage you to make a list of positive affirmations, and make them in the present tense. For instance " I am........." or " I can....." That way your conscious brain starts to believe what you tell it. Laminate the sayings, and put them up all over your home. You will become filled with their message. I do. Even more, you will be adding value to those who come over to your home. They too will become inspired.

Like the saying goes, you can't give birth to something if you haven't conceived it. Go ahead, conceive your new repositioned life!

Check www.doctorisabel.co.nz for the upcoming date of "Your PureLifestyle Cleanse" for your start to permanent weight loss.

Chapter 5. How to Block

In this section we will learn the technique of blocking out all thoughts that would hinder, your new re-created healthy self, from blossoming. But before we go any further, I want to congratulate you! Yes, you. Why? Please allow me to explain. Having a health goal should be something we all have and want to achieve. Unfortunately, we can't rely on hope or a magic pill to make us fit and healthy. We can't blame someone else for our bad health decisions either.

We all make choices in life, and we need to take responsibility for it AND, you have. To that I congratulate you. Strong work.

How do we make choices?

I realize that I have discussed earlier in this book, the importance of writing down your goals. But in all actuality, I want to re-emphasize this, and say it in a different way, because of it's importance in your success. Your success is important to me.

Here are the 3 steps to making a choice.

1. Have a goal. Having a goal makes you stronger, healthier and happier.

2. Write it down. By writing it down you are claiming that goal for yourself. The seed of that goal will germinate and take root in the subconscious soil of both your mind and your heart and produce fruit.

Let me give you a recent real life miracle illustration, in my life:

A mentor and friend of mine Dave Bradley, author of Build Your Team, Build Your Dream, told me 2 years ago that he was in the process of writing a book. I immediately thought to myself, "I have a book inside me that I want to write. "That is what happens when you are mentored by people of integrity and vision, you begin to mirror them. There was just one problem. I didn't write down my goal, to write a book. And so I really didn't mirror my mentor. It wasn't until Dave told me that his book was finished and he sent Michael and I a copy, in New Zealand, that it hit me. I still had the goal to write a book BUT I hadn't written my goal to write a book down. I woke up and wrote my goal down. Guess what? The next execution step appeared! Michael got an email from another one of our mentors Dr. John Maxwell, author of 73 books on ...wait for it.....wait for it......".A day about books and how to write a book", webinar in June 2012. And the rest is history. Can you see how the simple step of writing down your goal leads to the next step and then the next step and then...? Pretty cool isn't it.

3. Reward yourself. Once you have achieved your goal you need to reward yourself. You deserved it. I don't mean with food. Consider a massage, pedicure, new outfit, walking shoes, movie, etc.

If you don't reach your goal...it is ok...you just reset the goal. No big deal. Progress occurs with mistakes. If you aren't failing, then you aren't moving, you are stagnant and not growing. Consider a child learning to walk. The child falls. Do you tell it to stay down? I thinketh not. You brush off the dirt and help it back up. Well, the same philosophy applies to you. Help yourself back up and reset the goal my friend.

On to blocking:

To become your best you need to stop listening to the wrong voices. I am giving you permission to close the door or put another way, to place a block on toxic people in your life.

• Be allergic to negative people.

•

• Be allergic to negative self talk.

•

• Know your enemy, which is your negative thoughts.

Remember the picture of your mind and your heart that we talked about earlier? The top part is your conscious part, the part that you are aware of. The bottom part is the subconscious part, the part that you are not aware of. Consider the bottom part full of soil.

When a farmer plants his seeds, he prepares the ground. This is because he knows a great seed planted in soil full of weeds will not produce a great crop.

The same philosophy applies to your success. All your success begins in your mind. So lets get your soil ready for planting shall we? There are the components of your soil.

1. **Faith.** Faith is knowing you are created to be your best and do great things. Faith reminds us to be open to a greater power; God, higher force, The Almighty One, for the way to your goals. It is realizing that it is not all up to you. All you need to be is open, teachable, and motivated to receive direction. I love the way Ralph Waldo Trine explains faith:

"Faith is an invisible and invincible magnet, and attracts to it whatever it fervently desires and calmly and persistently expects" But ......you still need to put in the W O R K. Work is a good four letter word. Which leads us to the next component of your soil.

2. **Belief.** Belief is the work part of faith. Belief is active not passive. I can give you an example.

When I decided to become a doctor, I had the faith to do it. I also had to put in the work, which was me believing that I would become a doctor. For you it might be, you have faith that you will lose weight and become a sexy younger you. However that will require work. "Whoever does not doubt at all in his heart, but believes that what he says will take place it will be done for him" Mark 11:23. Yes, you just gotta believe your goals will occur.

3. **Weeds**. Every farmer has to make sure that he sprays for weeds. He knows that a great seed planted in soil full of weeds will not produce a great crop.

What kind of weeds are we talking about?

• Bitterness

• Unforgiveness

• Hatred

• Jealousy

• Greed

• Cynicism

• Doubt.

Be on the alert for these weeds. They will stop you dead in your tracks and you will never reach your goal. Ok, now we have our mind and heart's soil ready with faith and belief. And we have sprayed for weeds. Now let's take a step outside of our mind and heart, and see how we can protect our selves from the outside environment. Imagine a door. On one side of the door is you. On the other side, is the world. This door can open and close.

The world consists of people and people can say positive or negative things. We can either open the door to what they say or close the door. I want to encourage you to open the door if it is positive, but slam it shut if it is negative. You have that power. I call closing the door to a negative... "Blocking". You can say it under your breath. You don't have to shout it out, people might think your nuts.

People that love you dearly can say some negative statements, and not even know they said it. I will use my husband Michael as an example only to prove a point. Not to pick on him. He really is my rock.

I announced to Michael that I was going to start telling a joke before I start all my public speaking engagements. I had seen other public speakers do it and found it fun. Michael's response was "Babe, you aren't good at telling jokes." Immediately in my head I said "Block". He didn't know I did it. I just did it. Now I know that Michael loves me and would do anything for me, but my point is even people that are close to you can say negative things. It is our responsibility to block those statements from access into our brain and heart.

Just shut the door. Just block it.

So access was denied and I went on to learn how to tell a joke. Now before every speaking engagement, I crack a joke, get the audience smiling and away we go. I love it!

Ch.6 Your Mastermind Team

When you have a dream or a goal you can start small, but don't start alone. In this chapter I will reveal to you who is on my mastermind team to help me succeed in reaching my dreams.

Before we start I need to prepare you.

You may think I am a little weird with what I am about to share with you, but that's ok. I would prefer you think that I am weird, than just a normal person. Being normal is nothing to brag about. There just is nothing creative in being normal. Plus being normal is not healthy. Take a look out there in the world and see what normal is. It just is not good.

I was reading an amazing book by Napoleon Hill called The Laws of Success. It took me about 16 months to complete it, because I read and applied one chapter per month. Mr. Hill helped me expand on a concept my mother taught me as a child, the concept of angels. Angels are very much a part of my invisible Mastermind team, and the Leader of my mastermind team is God. In the bible it says "For He shall give His Angels charge over you, to keep you in all your ways. In their hands they shall bear you up, so you don't dash your foot against a stone." Psalm 91:11-12. That is just so thoughtful of God to give us angels that will help us hydroplaning over the rough patches of our life so that we don't even scratch our feet.

Let me introduce you to my 11 Angels, each with their own unique place on my path to success:

Patience. Patience teaches me to have composure while I wait. I am naturally a very impatient person. My husband Michael on the other hand is very patient. It is very helpful to see patience in action by looking at the way he handles rough spots. And it is great to have my angel Patience help me be more like Michael.

Joy. I call my joy angel, "Shasta", because we use to have a dog with that name. Shasta had the spirit of joy in her always, no matter what. Nothing could ever take her joy away. Shasta teaches me to enjoy this journey, not dread it.

Health. I call my health angel, "Doc". Doc goes to work when I go to sleep. If I am sick or in pain before I go to bed, then I ask him to please get to work. And when I get up, I am feeling better and stronger and healed. Most of the time. Sometimes he has to work a double or triple shift on me.

Wisdom. Guides me to make right choices

Financial Prosperity. Helps me do the following;

• not over spend

- set goals

- invest

- have abundant thinking.

Peace of mind. Peace sings this song that you may know. I'll sing you a line....."Everything is gonna be all right , yea...cuz that's the seeds I sow...Wowowo, wowowo, wowowo wo" How was that? Peace reminds me that all I have to do is, trust God and do right. Simple enough.

Hope and Faith. These two are together because you can't have one without the other. Hope tells me to never, ever, ever give up. Hope also coaches me to expect better and better comes. Faith reminds me to worry about nothing and pray about everything.

Love and Romance. This pair that cannot exist without the other. Love tells me to always believe the best and wish well for my enemies. Love also helps me develop love for ALL of humanity, because a negative attitude towards others will never bring me success. Romance adds the right mood to the whole project.

Roaming Ambassador. I call her " Gwenie". She was another dog we used to have, but we had to put her down because she was very ill with liver cancer. Gwenie does everything else the other angels don't, like finds me a good parking spot, and lets me know about good clothing sales.

There you have my invisible mastermind team. They are priceless and always on call for me. I am grateful for my mom and Mr. Hill for talking to me about them.

In closing I want to leave you with this

Some people have a dream but no team--their dream is impossible.

Some people have a dream and are building a team--their dream has potential.

Some people have a dream and a great team--their dream is inevitable.

-Dr. John Maxwell

Part 5: Effective Exercise

It's Like Brushing Your teeth and paying taxes...we have to do it.
<><><><>

Ch.1 Quick Facts for Your Back Pocket

Who loves to exercise? Unfortunately it's something we have to do, just like brushing our teeth, taking a shower, and paying taxes.

Exercise can dig up some bad thoughts like; being embarrassed, painful thoughts because you only do it when you have to lose weight. Maybe you were always the last one to be picked for the team, or it brings up the notion of pain, because of the lactic-acid build up it caused. Regardless we need to shake that bootie whether your young, old, or old-young.

I like to focus on the positives. Here the benefits.

- Controls weight

- Promotes maximum bone density...so they don't break as easily

- Strengthens and tones

- Enhances flexibility

- Boosts energy

- Promotes better sleep

- Improves quality of life

- Combats health conditions and diseases

- Improves mood

- lowers blood sugar

- lowers blood pressure

- Promotes social well-being by improving self-confidence and the ability to interact socially with peers.

   In addition, it was demonstrated at the University of Colorado, that modest exercise can even help prevent colds. This study found people who participated in a daily exercise program were less likely to get sick after stressful situations. The bottom line is that we need to change our attitude about exercise. If you are still struggling with the concept of exercise, then I encourage you to change what you are saying to yourself.

Remember if we can change our words we can change our life.

Start by saying:

- I am becoming a better me.

- I feel great when I exercise.

- I can do it!

- day by day in every way I am getting stronger and stronger.

- I may not be where I want to be, but at least I am not where I used to be.

- make exercise a priority.

   When you reach a goal, remember to reward yourself with something nice like clothes, movie, hot bath, message etc.

Hope that helps.

Ch.2 Interval Training

There are three parts to effective exercise:

1. Interval training

2. Resistance training

3. Rest

Interval training is another term used to replace cardio training. Studies have indicated that exercise with a burst component to it, is more effective in helping people lose weight. Especially the belly fat. Over-exercising can actually make us fat. When I heard this, I really felt like my brain had been scrambled. How can this occur?

Remember back in the earlier chapter this following diagram

You can see how stress raises your cortisol levels and in the end the body stores fat. This is what happens if we stress our bodies. This really happened to me. Michael and I would religiously wake up at 5am to go to bike spinning class, you make know it as RPM. It is a full on bike session for 60 minutes. The goal was to burn calories. We burned calories all right. We also gained weight and not the good muscle kind. We were at it for one and half years, three times a week.

Until I came across the diagram above. This made me realize, that though we were burning calories and sweating up a storm, we were also stressing our bodies out. This caused cortisol to be increased, which resulted in storage of fat.

What did I do next? I slept in! A 5 am start in the gym is just nasty. Next I started to add interval training and the weight keeps on coming off, even at my tender age of 52 years young.

The back bone of interval training is simple.

- 5-10 warm up

- 1:2 ratio of a work out

- 5-20 min of the 1:2 ratio

- 5 min cool down

- 2-3 times a week

For instance 30 sec. hard at an exercise, then recovery is 60 sec., 6-8 reps of this. Ideas could be biking, jogging, rowing, walking, swimming, jump rope, stairs,

Studies have found you can boost your metabolism, burn more calories all day long and lose more weight by exercising less....all I can say to that is a big Yahoo!

You also are getting another benefit by doing interval training. Your body is not experiencing oxidative stress, therefore you won't age like the other exercises that stress your body.

Ch. 3 Resistance Training

Resistance training has a different goal. Where interval training increases your metabolism to burn fat, resistance training has a different goal. It strengthens your muscles which helps you burn fat all day long. This is called "Afterburn", which is burning fat while you are resting. It also keeps you looking and acting young.

You read right. Having more muscle makes your body younger. Conversely, having more fat is a stress on your poor body and it ages you, real fast. Fat ages you, puts a stress load on your system AND increase inflammation which leads to chronic disease such as Hypertension, Diabetes Type 2, Heart Disease, certain Cancers and Alzheimer's Disease. Having more muscle melts away the fat and you become a lean fat burning machine instead of a fat storing machine.

Women do not need to do heavier weights, just the lighter weights. Rest assured, women do not bulk up because they don't have testosterone. Men, on the other hand, have testosterone and therefore bulk up with muscle. Do this 20-30 minutes per session, 2-3 times a week, and you will become "Mighty fine scenery"

Question: How do we lose weight?

Answer: With both interval and resistance training.

Women-Just the facts.

Remember I am just the messenger so please don't "shoot the messenger"

1. According to the American Journal of Preventative Medicine -A married women who has 1 baby gains an average of 20 pounds (9 kg) over 10 years.

2. For every child we have, increases our rate of obesity by 7% over our lifetime. If we have 3 children our risk of obesity increase by 21% (Duke University Medical Center)

Why does this happen? Pregnancy causes an increase in insulin production, which results in accumulation of fat.

3. Menopausal women have an average weight gain of 12 pounds (5 kg) within 8 years after menopause. Fat burning decreases 32% due to a decrease in estrogen according to a study in the International Journal of obesity.

 All the more reason for us ladies to do interval and resistance training to stay younger and sexy.

Men - Just the facts

Same applies here...remember I am just the messenger. (big smiley face just for you)

As you age, there is a lack of testosterone. That is the hormone, that makes you all muscular and sexy. With aging there is a natural tendency for that muscle to become fat. That fat likes to accumulate around the belly area, which is very dangerous. Where there is belly fat, there is an increased risk of a heart attack.

And for I also recommend interval and resistance training

What about the last step, Rest?

And lastly we want to rest...Ahhh. Rest between workouts. You won't get results if you don't. Muscles actually grow when they are resting. If you don't rest and over train then your body will get tired and stressed, which leads to decrease energy, increase sickness and oxidative stress(you will age faster)

Exercise Guide

1. Interval Training

- 5-10 minutes warm-up

- 1:2 ratio, for example 30 seconds hard out (puffing hard) , 60 seconds slow pace (don't stop just slow down)

- 6-8 repetitions

- Running, running up stairs, biking, jogging,walking,rowing, swimming, jumping rope.

- Approximately 20 minutes of 1:2 ratio. If you can only do 5 minutes that's fantastic. Pace yourself to get to 20 minutes. You will get there.

- 5 minute cool down

- 2-3 times a week

2. Resistance Training

- lift some type of weight

- 20-30 minutes per day

- 2-3 times a week

3. Rest.

- Alternate Interval with resistance through out the week with at least one full day off of everything.

- Maybe on your rest day you take a 45 minute walk.

Part 6: Sugar, Obesity, and Our Future   <><><><><>

Chapter 1. My Journey with Sugar

I want to begin this chapter with a story.

A mother brought her child to see Gandhi and asked him, "Please tell my child to stop eating sugar." Gandhi said, "Bring her back in 3 days". Three days later the mother brings her child back to him and asked. "I am confused, why did you tell me to come back in three days?" Gandhi said," because three days ago I was eating sugar."

I tell you this story because I know how hard it is to give away sugar. I was a sugar junkie, remember I was the doc who had a bag of skittles and coffee for a strong start to my morning. Society has a sugar addiction, and we have an overweight problem. People are bulging out of their clothes. Especially the kids.

So how did I break off my love affair with sugar. It was a decision I made when I realized that I was being tricked to eat more sugar. If we eat a low fat diet then the fat is replaced with sugar and salt. I to, believed, that in order to be healthy I needed to consume a low fat diet. Guess what happens when you take the fat out of food? It tastes like cardboard. You also don't feel satisfied after eating. You see, eating fat is satisfying. In other words it fills you up. When I also learned that excess sugar gets stored as fat, the alarm bells went off. Oh it wasn't pretty in our house. I have two teenage daughters and my husband who were also addicted to sugar. The problem was they didn't realize it. My mother has always described me as a pioneer and courageous. I went through our cupboards and refrigerator and began reading labels. The more I read, the madder I got, and the fuller the trash bin got.

I have a saying "Waking up is very painful." It is painful to face reality because we get comfortable in our routines. The routine of going to do groceries, and buying the same cereal week after week after week. Until one day you wake up, begin reading the label, and find within the first 5 ingredients, is some form of sugar. I just got mad when I realized, I was poisoning my family and affecting their health. However before I was able to "talk the talk", I had to "walk the talk". So, I went on a sugar fast. It was ugly!

I did not allow one drop of any type of sugar past my lips for one month. The only thing sweet into my mouth was 1-2 low GI pieces of fruit per day such as:

• grapefruit

• kiwi

• coconut

• strawberries

• apple

• avocado

• any berry

• plum

• green grapes

• cherries

It is mind blowing to taste the natural sweetness in fruit.

The withdrawals consisted of those, any addict experiences when they come off their drug of choice. Sugar is the same. Headaches, sugar, and carb craving, joint pain, fatigue, loss of clarity of thinking, and low moods. The only withdrawal I was spared was the sweating. But the good news is, it goes away and so does some weight. I bet you are wondering if I ever eat sugar. That's like asking me if the pope is catholic? There are times, when I just go for it and have sugar. I am a human being. The difference now is it doesn't go on day after day, year after year.

Back to my family. After my month of withdrawals, I had the right heart attitude to deal with my family's sugar withdrawal. Then I put them on a sugar detox. How? I just stopped bringing sugared foods into the home. No more ice cream, cereal, tomato sauce, cookies, cakes, jams, lunch box snacks, chips, sauces, on and on and on. I am glad to say we are still all alive and living under the same roof. My family really loved the weight loss that goes with it to. Yes, we do have treats, but very limited. After all, I want to stay alive.

If you are the person who brings the food into the home, I encourage you to do as Gandhi did and stop eating sugar. Then you will better understand and better guide your family through the tough times of removing sugar from their life, well at least 80%.

Below is a list of places sugar hides. I know I have shown this in a previous chapter but I really believe having this information will add value to your life and those you come in contact with.

Places where sugar hides:

- Agave syrup or agave sugar; Yes , agave has a low GI profile, however what it does is far worse than raise insulin levels. It raises your triglyceride levels, trigger inflammation and damage your liver.

- Barley malt

- Beet sugar

- Brown sugar

- Buttered syrup

- Cane juice crystals

- Cane sugar

- Caramel

- Corn syrup

- Corn syrup solids

- Confectioner's sugar
- Carob syrup
- Castor sugar
- Date sugar
- Demerara sugar
- Dextran
- Dextrose
- Diastatic malt
- Diatese
- Dried fruit (high GI and is all just concentrated sugar)
- Ethyl Maltol
- Fructose
- Fruit juice
- Fruit juice concentrate
- Galactose
- Glucose
- Glucose solids
- Golden sugar
- Golden syrup
- Grape sugar
- High-fructose corn syrup (HFCS)
- Sugar of maize
- Honey
- Icing sugar
- Invert sugar

- Lactose

- Maltodextrin

- Maltose

- Malt syrup

- Maple syrup

- Molasses

- Muscovado sugar

- Panocha

- Raw sugar

- Refiner's sugar

- Rice syrup

- Sorbitol

- Sorghum syrup

- Sucrose

- Sugar

- Treacle

- Turbinado sugar

- Yellow sugar

- and finally anything ending in "ose" is sugar.

You now have your Phd. in "sugar disguises." Now the question arises, "What can I use as a sweetener?" I always recommend Stevia. Stevia is a plant from the sunflower family and is 300 times sweeter than sugar. Stevia is a low GI food and if you need something as a sweetener then stevia is your best option. This is what we use in our family. I personally prefer the Stevia drops, as I can control the sweetness more readily, as opposed to the powder.

I promise you that once you remove all of the above from your life, the foods that you do eat, will taste sweet. You can do this. Plus, as a bonus, you will instantly loose some weight.

Ch. 2 The Bitter Truth

Dr. Lustig is a pediatrician, at The University of San Francisco, USA. He has put together a lecture called, "The Bitter Truth" which I encourage you to view on You-tube.

He is on a mission to end obesity and diabetes in our youth. I am in complete agreement with this.

The old thinking was a patient goes to the their doctor to lose weight. The doctor then gives the following equation:

Eat less + Eat a low fat diet + Exercise more = This will result in weight loss

When the patient comes back without losing weight the doctor thinks, they are lazy gluttons with no will power. Again the poor patient gets the same prescription but this time with a diet pill:

Diet pill + Eat less + Eat a low fat diet + Exercise more

Perhaps they lose a bit of weight when the diet pill is added, but long term the weight comes back with a few more pounds on top of it. The argument that children are lazy gluttons just doesn't stand either. No child chooses to be obese. They just eat what they are given. No one chooses to be obese for that matter.

I have been a doctor for 22 years and all I can say is "This does not work!"

Yes, we are eating more, but that is not the cause of 2/3 of America, UK, Australia, and NZ being overweight; AND of those 1/3 are obese.

We need to rethink the equation and unlearn what we have learned.

Put most eloquently by Mark Twain; "Education consists mainly of what we have unlearned"

In the past we have focused on BMI as an indicator of weight. Where

• less than 19 BMI = underweight

• 20-25 BMI = healthy

• 26-29 BMI = Overweight

• greater than 30 = Obese

We need to unlearn this and relearn the new .

The new measurement is our waist size. Now the goal is to have your waist size be less than half of your height.

For instance if you are 170 cm, then ideally your waist should be less than 85 cm. Alternatively, if you are 72 inches (6 ft.) then your waist circumference should be 36 inches or less.

A new study by Dr. Amen of the Amen Clinics in USA, states:

"An increase size of your waist leads to a decrease in the size of your brain."

So the bigger your waist, the smaller your brain. Now that should scare everyone into loosing those unhealthy love handles.

Does diet and exercise work? No. People gain weight when they exercise. Remember, when the body is stressed, cortisol is released which stores fat.

People have been telling me they are exercising and they don't loose weight. That is exactly right. If we exercise past a certain point, it stresses the body and the body starts to store fat for future energy. We even have an epidemic of obese six month olds and they don't exercise. So exercise is not the answer.

Looking at behavior

What makes us obese?

There are many reasons why there is so much obesity all around us in the western world. What surrounds us has the most impact.

- Food is available to us 24 hours per day 7 days a week.

- Food tastes really good. Food companies put in **food enhancers** to make food smell and taste good. I had a patient go into Burger king for a meal. He said it "tasted good when I am eating it , but boy it is painful when it lands." The reason he was in to see me was because he had diarrhea the next day and needed an off work certificate.

- There are more TV food commercials. Count the amount of food commercials you see next time you are watching TV. The average child sees 10,000 ads for junk food on TV in one year. American Idol has judges with Coke cups in front of them.

- Grocery stores have all the sugar products on the lower shelves. This is purposely done for the viewing of our children.

- There is something in our diet called **High Fructose Corn Syrup (HFCS),** which we will address shortly.

- In 1980 we were told to decrease fat and increase our sugar consumption by eating more carbs. We now know this didn't work. As I have mentioned before, when you take the fat out of food you need to make it taste better, and that was accomplished by adding HFCS.

Bottom line is we are influenced by what we see and smell.

Ch. 3 High Fructose Corn Syrup.

In the past 30 years, the sugar calories we consume, from high fructose corn syrup (HFCS) have increased from 0% to 66%. This sadly is due to the consumption of soft drinks and other sweetened beverages. We also know that liquid calories in the form of sugar, packs on the weight.

What is HFCS?

HFCS is an industrial food product, which is far from being considered natural or for that matter a whole food. It is extracted from corn stalks through a chemical process, which makes it sweeter than sugar. It is also cheaper, and as a result, is used more readily than sugar.

What does it do to our body?

This compound is rapidly absorbed into our bloodstream and sent to our liver. Once in the liver, a reaction called lipogenesis (the production of fats like triglycerides and cholesterol) occurs. Your liver gets taxed from over working and this is the major cause of liver damage, also known as fatty liver. In addition, because it is so rapidly absorbed, there is a spike in our insulin. Because of these two features of HFCS there is an increase in appetite, weight gain, diabetes, heart disease, dementia that we know of to date.

In addition it affects our gut. In our intestine there are these connections between the intestinal cells called "tight junctions." They have one main purpose and that is to allow nutrients in, and prevent bacteria and other not so healthy food compounds through. If the bacteria where to get through these "tight junctions" then this triggers an immune and body wide inflammation response. What is interesting about HFCS, is that it does just that by, punching holes in the intestinal lining of the gut. The problem is, it allows the enemy in, and all war breaks out in your gut. You may have heard of this as referred to a "Leaky Gut Syndrome". HFCS is one the things that make this occur.

What does HFCS contain?

An FDA researcher asked corn producers to ship a barrel of high fructose corn syrup to her so that she could test for contaminants. Her repeated requests were denied until she claimed she represented a newly created soft drink company. She was then promptly shipped a big vat of HFCS, which was used in a study that showed that HFCS often contains toxic levels of mercury, due to the chlor-alkali products used in it's manufacturing.

I wish to emphasize something here. The companies that produce HFCS often say in TV ads that HFCS is exactly like sugar. I want you to realize one thing: Poisoned sugar, like that created in the production of HFCS, is certainly not natural.

Real sugar consists of glucose and fructose. When HFCS is placed through a chemical analyzer, strange peaks show up that do not coincide with the normal glucose and fructose peaks. We don't really know what it is and the producers of HFCS don't really want to share their recipe. And to think that 20% of the western world is consuming this poison, is not only disturbing, but frightening.

Do we need HFCS in our diets?

If you go to the friendly and happy looking websites by the corn industry www.cornsugar.com and www.sweetsurprise.com, they say they have the same position as the nutritional experts. The only problem is they are mis-quoting the nutritional experts.

Barry M. Popkins, PhD. Professor, Department of Nutrition, University of North Carolina at Chapel Hill, has published widely on the dangers of sugar-sweetened drinks and their contribution to our obesity epidemic. In a review of HFCS in the American Journal of Clinical Nutrition, he explains the mechanism by which free fructose may contribute to obesity. He states that:

The digestion, absorption, and metabolism of fructose differ from those of glucose. Hepatic metabolism of fructose favors de novo lipogenesis. In addition, unlike glucose, fructose does not stimulate insulin secretion or enhance leptin production. Because insulin and leptin act as key afferent signals in the regulation of food intake and body weight (to control appetite), this suggests that dietary fructose may contribute to increased energy intake and weight gain. Furthermore, calorically sweetened beverages may enhance caloric overconsumption.

Dr. Popkin concludes by saying that "the increase in consumption of HFCS has a temporal relation to the epidemic of obesity, and the overconsumption of HFCS in calorically sweetened beverages may play a role in the epidemic of obesity."

The corn industry takes his comments out of context to support their position, that "all sugar is the same."

Here is a biochemistry lesson about cane sugar and HFCS in a nutshell.

• Cane sugar is sucrose and it is composed of 50% fructose and 50% glucose.

   Sucrose (cane sugar) = 50% fructose + 50% glucose

• HFCS is different. HFCS is made up of 45% fructose and 55% glucose

   HFCS = 45% fructose + 55% glucose

The point here is glucose is sweeter than fructose, so HFCS is sweeter than naturally occurring cane sugar because it has a higher percentage of glucose. So their quote that "all sugar is the same" is false.

HFCS is not "a naturally occurring" substance in nature. HFCS is extracted from corn stalks and processed in a mystery spoken about in Michael Pollan's book called "The Omnivores Dilemma".

True, large doses of any sugar is harmful, and in the end it might be the pharmacologic doses of any type of sugar that kill you. But the biochemistry of cane sugar and HFCS and how it affects our absorption, our appetite, and our metabolism are different. And Dr. Popkin knows that.

Is HFCS a marker of poor quality, nutrient poor and a disease -creating food product?

Simple answer is Yes. If you find "High-fructose corn syrup" or the terms: "corn sugar" or "sugar of maize" on the label, you can be sure it is not a whole, real, fresh food, full of fiber, vitamins and minerals.

In summary, I highly recommend for you to reduce your overall consumption of sugar all together. However more importantly removing this one simple dietary change (cutting out HFCS), will radically reduce your health risks and improve your overall health.

" To be forewarned is to be forearmed "

Ch 4 Is Diet Food Making You Fat?

When the low fat revolution began, along with it came the use of artificial sweeteners. So then everyone was told to eat low fat foods, and drink diet drinks. That's what I was taught in medical school. That was all the information I had to offer my patients. I have learned differently, and I want to share with you some very interesting information regarding artificial sweeteners.

To start with, we need to understand why we eat.

What drives the desire to eat?

Eating food gives us satisfaction and shares in the same brain circuitry with other pleasurable activities such as sex and drug administration. We call this food reward.

Food reward has two roads. One to the brain, and the other away from the brain.

The first road to the brain, is called the sensory road. When we eat there are signals that go to our brain to tell us we just ate something. Then there is another road that leaves the brain to tell our gut that we have received enough food and we are full. This is call called the postingestive road.

When rats are deprived of food, then given a choice between glucose (which has 15 calories per teaspoon, in it) versus saccharin (which has no calories), they preferred the glucose. It appears that that the artificial sweetener does not send a message along the postingestive pathway to the gut telling it "you are full."

In another study at Purdue University's Ingestive Behavior Research Center, reported that relative to rats that ate yogurt sweetened with glucose (which has calories), rats given yogurt sweetened with 0- calorie saccharin later;

• consumed more calories

• gained more weight

• put on more body fat

• and didn't make up for it by cutting back on consumption.

Put more succinctly in the Yale Journal of Biology and Medicine, "lack of completed satisfaction, likely because of the failure to activate the postingestive component, further fuels the food seeking." So those that use artificial sweeteners are never full and keep eating.

I realize that this is all done on rats and not on humans, but the findings match emerging evidence that people who drink more diet drinks are at higher risk for obesity. They are also at risk developing metabolic syndrome, which is a collection of medical problems such as abdominal fat, high blood pressure, and insulin resistance that put people at risk for heart disease and diabetes.

So if you are thinking that diet soft drinks are the answer to weight loss. I strongly encourage you to think again. Evidence is mounting that they lead to weight gain rather then weight loss. Those who consume diet drinks regularly have a 200 percent increased risk of weight gain and a 67 percent increase risk of diabetes.

A study of over 400 people found that those who drank two diet sodas per day had five times the increase in waist circumference as those who did not drink soda.

What are the names of artificial sweeteners?

• Nutrasweet

• Splenda

• Acesulfame potassium Ace K

• Aspartame

• Cyclamate

• Isomalt

• Saccharin

• Sucralose

• Alitame

• Neohesperidine dihydrochalcone

• Aspartame-acesulfame salt

• Sorbitol

• Maltitol

If you need something sweet, then I recommend stevia. As mentioned in Chapter 1; My Journey with sugar, stevia comes from the sunflower family, is low GI and is 300x sweeter than sugar. I personally don't like the aftertaste, however it is the safest natural sweetener out there.

Ch. 5 What is Diabesity

When we go to the doctor and have our blood checked, they normally do a screening test to check for type 2 diabetes. This test, currently, is called a HgA1c (hemaglobin A1c). If it is under a certain number, then you are told that you don't have type 2 diabetes. However if it is over a certain number you are told you now have type 2 diabetes.

The problem with this approach is that type 2 diabetes doesn't happen over a month or a year. It actually starts much earlier, years, even decades. There is a journey one goes on before they are given the dreaded diagnosis of type 2 diabetes.

The various markers before one is told they have diabetes is given different names such as:

• Insulin Resistance

• Metabolic Syndrome

• Syndrome X

• Obesity

• Pre-diabetes

• Adult onset diabetes

• Type 2 diabetes All of these are essentially one problem and the cause that drives all of these conditions are essentially the same.

According to Mark Hyman MD, author of The Blood Sugar Solution, he states a more comprehensive term to describe the continuum from optimal blood sugar to insulin resistance to full blown diabetes is **diabesity.** In short, diabesity is the road one is on and the final destination is type 2 diabetes.

Diabesity (mild insulin resistance > obesity > type 2 diabetes) is the single biggest global health epidemic of our time. It is the leading cause of chronic disease such as heart disease, stroke, dementia, and cancer. The point we want to bring home to you is these are all preventable diseases. You don't have to have them.

We know what the root of the problem is. "As physicians, we are trained to offer medication or surgery to solve diabetes (and disease in general), when the real causes include poor-quality diet, nutritional deficiencies, hormonal imbalances, allergens, microbes, digestive imbalances, toxins, cellular energy problems, and stress. We think that treating the risk factors, such as high blood pressure, high blood sugar, cholesterol, with medications will help. But we don't learn how to identify and treat the *real* causes of disease", says Dr. Hyman.

We need to ask the most important questions which are;

- why is your blood sugar high?

- why is your blood pressure high?

- why is your cholesterol high?

The bottom line is, type 2 diabetes and elevated blood sugar, blood pressure, and cholesterol are symptoms that result from problems with diet, lifestyle, and environmental toxins. By 2020, 1 in 2 people will have diabesity, and 90% will not know it, because it is not being taught in medical schools. Doctors don't even know how to test for it.

This is not just an adult problem, this is a childhood tragedy. We are now seeing eight-year-old children with type 2 diabetes, which in the past was called "adult onset diabetes". Fifteen year olds with type 2 diabetes, are having strokes, and twenty-five-year olds are requiring cardiac bypass. This is shocking. This is the first generation of children in history that will live sicker and die younger than their parents.

"From 1983 to 2008, the number of people in the world with diabetes increased sevenfold, from 35 to 240 million. In just three years, from 2008 to 2011, we added another 110 million diabetics to our global population" states Dr. Hyman.

He adds and I agree, " Shouldn't the main question we ask be, why is this happening, instead of what new drug can we find to treat it? Our approach must be novel, innovative, and widely applicable at low cost across all borders." Too many billions of dollars have been spent trying to find the right "drug cure".

What I hope I have done is shown you that the solution is right under our nose...our mouth and what we put into it. This is a lifestyle and environmental disease and will not be cured by medication.

Lets wake up, lets rise up and take back our health for our sake and more importantly for our children's life.

Ch.6   What Can We Do?

One of the most important take home messages for you today is to know that you are in control, if you choose to be in control. If you do, then you can experience what it is like to feel clean, full of energy and have that glow that healthy people exude. If you choose not to take control of your health, because it is too hard, then I recommend you go to the hospital and volunteer and care for those who chose likewise. I pray that someday you wake up.

The most challenging step most people express is, giving up sugar. The reason you want to give up all types of sugar is because it spikes your insulin. Type 2 diabetes is due to to much insulin being around. Now the question we want to ask is WHY is there so much insulin around? The answer is because there is so much sugar around. So lets get rid of the root of the problem seen in type 2 diabetes...sugar. Remember, when there is to much insulin around , then insulin will store sugar away as fat.....especially belly fat. You want to avoid that.

Give yourself about a month to detox from sugar and you will see your waist circumference decrease, your weight comes off and your energy levels increase. Promise.

6 Simple Steps for Kicking Sugar Cravings.

1. Avoid sugar foods.

Sugar and processed foods can be as addictive as heroin. Eating sugar artificially stimulates a region in your brain called the "nucleus accumbens" which produces **dopamine, the pleasure hormone**. Soon dopamine levels drop and we start to feel "flat" or a bit down. So we grab for more sugar, and round and round and up and down we go. We crave this pleasant, feel-good emotion again........**so sugar leads to addiction.**

2. Boost your serotonin.

Serotonin is known as your "happy hormone", and it can be increased by;

a. eating a low GI diet as explained in Part 1 Chapter 4 called What do I eat doc?

b. 8-9 hours of good sleep

c. regular exercise

When you have sufficient serotonin, you are less likely to crave sweets.

3. Use Stevia to satisfy your sweet tooth.

Stevia, as mentioned before is a natural sweetener, no calories, won't spike your blood sugar levels, and is 300 times sweeter than sugar. It does have an after taste though. Stevia comes in powder and liquid form and can be purchased at a health food store.

4. Drink plenty of water.

Sometimes when you think you are hungry, you are actually thirsty. Try water with 5 drops of stevia and a squeeze of lemon, lime, or orange.

5. Keep your blood sugars stable.

To avoid dips in your blood sugar eat a combination of a carbohydrate, fat and protein every 4 hours at each sitting. Try a celery stick or wholemeal cracker with organic almond butter or organic peanut butter for a snack.

6. Have plenty of vegetables ready.

Green veggies help boost your energy and reduce cravings for sugar and processed foods. Have some always chopped up and ready to eat in the refrigerator. Try juicing your veggies for a super-charged nutrient boost. Juicing gives you a super fantastic way to add life giving nutrients and detoxifying plant chlorophyll to your blood stream.

What doesn't work

We also need to look at what just doesn't work. In the past we have tried to have public campaigns and government guidelines to help. For instance warning on product labels such as cigarettes and still people continue to smoke. Or school based education programs regarding alcohol abuse. We still have an incredible amount of binge drinking amongst our teenagers.

Why they don't work is very simply because our brains have been hijacked by advertisement. For every logical advertisement about the dangers of cigarettes and alcohol there are two to three times more showing how sexy and cool it is to drink and smoke. The youth want to be accepted. Guess who wins?

What I do know, is this. Sugar is addictive like nicotine, alcohol, cannabis, morphine, amphetamine, cocaine and heroin. And we have a food war upon on us. What is good for the food companies, which is producing cheap, non-food that makes a good profit, is bad for us. I don't recommend this but the message is clear... If you want to make money, then invest in fast food.

Addiction is not only a personal responsibility but also a social and governmental responsibility. Just saying "No" is not the answer. It is bigger than this. It would be fantastic is we could make a drug to stop a sugar addiction but there is no possible way from a chemical point of view.

Are you familiar with the Pottenger experiment with the cats? This is an old experiment that has been repeated multiple times. Pottenger fed cats raw food and dead food. After eating dead food the cats were extinct in four generations. The raw food cats were thriving. They had great hair and skin. What do people eat today? They are eating dead food.

Another thing I know is ...people don't want to be obese. Children don't want to be obese. It happens because their bodies are starved for real, whole, nutrient dense food, so they continue to eat hoping to feed their hungry bodies. Sadly enough, they just keep getting dead nutrient deficient food.

What needs to work

Since we are influenced by what we see and hear, there needs to be controls on advertising. Just look around us and we can see the toys at McDonalds is one of the ways the kids are advertised to. We need to be more like Norway, Sweden, UK and 46 other countries around the world that ban advertising to children.

A taxation such as a "Soda Tax" would also help to decrease consumption. Just like there is a cigarette tax in certain parts of the world, we know that increasing the cost of a product decreases its use.

We should also see fast food chains have to pay a certain amount yearly to the medical cost of a country. They are, contributing to the tsunami of obesity and diabetes, so they should help pay for its affects. If the food chain has a product that takes away health then it needs to be held accountable. This will help pay the enormous costs of obesity and the chronic diseases associated with it.

On the other hand if a food chain adds value to a country, then the opposite should occur. They are given a tax break. This approach would encourage other entrepreneurs to create food companies that help heal the world. They would be adding to the solution instead of adding to the problem.

There should be restrictions on consumption. For instance, why are corner stores a few meters from schools? Maybe there should be a restriction where there are no sales of sugar products from 3-6pm.

We at Purelifestyle are in the process of forming health teams that teach and guide schools and corporations about nutrition. What I have found is that everyone needs help on the rules of the body and what it needs. When we can affect one person, one school, one corporation then they will affect their world.

Like the saying goes:

"One can put a thousand to flight, two can put ten thousand to flight." Deuteronomy 32:30

Can you envision what 200 can do? If our teams can work with the CEO of a home, which is usually the one who buys the food, then they will change the world of their home for this generation and generations to come. It all starts with one. Just look at what Mother Teresa and Gandhi have done.

I am looking for big thinkers to join forces with. If you have any new ideas, please contact me at:

info@doctorisabel.co.nz

Check www.doctorisabel.co.nz for the upcoming date of "Your PureLifestyle Cleanse" for your start to permanent weight loss.

Part 7: Putting It All Together

Living a Super-Fantastic Life w/o Disease <><><>

Chapter 1. Eating Your Medicine

We have been lead to believe that if we eat whatever we want, we can counteract that with exercising. There is nothing further from the truth. There are 32 years old who did just that, and are having heart attacks.

You have come this far and you are now well equipped to walk your journey back to health. There are just a few basics you need to keep in mind.

First, your medicine is at the end of your fork. You truly are what you eat. If you eat dead food, you will feel dead. If you eat live food, you will feel alive. It is as simple as that.

If you can buy organic food go for it. If you can't, I understand. Then your next step is to make sure you wash your fruits and vegetables in one part white vinegar, to ten parts water. Swish around and rinse with water. This will help remove the pesticides that reside underneath the skin.

Second, drink your water. Your body is 75% water. There are so many times my patients come in and say "I feel so tired." When I ask how much water they drink, they will tell me, one to two pump bottles. That's about 500-750 ml of water. The goal is to drink at least 30 ml of water for every kg of weight. Or if you are working in pounds, that comes out to 1 ounce of water for every pound of weight.

70 kg person x 30 ml/kg = 2.1 liters of water per day

154 lb person x 1 ounce/lb = 154 ounces or 1 gallon of water per day

Make sure you don't drink it all in one sitting as that is dangerous. Divide the water portions into 1/3 and consume through out the day.

Third, follow the food pyramid chart that you have in Part 1 Chapter 2. This will become second nature to you after a while. You also have a list of low to high GI foods in Part 1 Chapter 4 What do I eat doc?

"The best way to break a bad habit is to replace it with a good on

You can do it. I know you can.

Chapter 2. Maximizing Your Health with Supplementation

Several of my patients ask me why they need vitamins and supplementation if they are already eating real, whole foods. Great question.

Supplements help fill in any gaps in your daily eating, when you are unable to get your requirements of micronutrients. Additionally, if we lived in a world that was;

• free of toxins

• we ate only 100% real food

• were stress free

• exercised regularly

• relaxed when we need to relax

• slept 8-9 hours every night

• drank our required amount of water

• and had good strong healthy relationships,

then I could responsibly say to you that you don't need vitamins and supplements. However, that is not the world we live in.

Here is a basic plan of what my family and myself take. I personally have a few more on top of this for my specific needs.

Multivitamin/Multimineral

Many multivitamins/multiminerals offer a broad spectrum formula, ideal for everyday use to support a balanced diet. However, not all contain the following, so make sure you are getting these:

- **Zinc** and **selenium** help to support a healthy immune system

- **Vitamin B** assists with healthy brain function and energy production.

- **Folic acid** to assist in the maintenance of a healthy cardiovascular system and maintain normal homocysteine levels. Homocysteine is a marker of cardiovascular health.

Omega-3 Fatty Acid

I can't say enough about the importance of eating good fats, and Omega-3's are the king among healthy fats.

Your body needs the right type of fats, and without them your body just breaks down. Every single cell in your body is made up of essential fats. Fats make up the wall of every single cell in your precious glorious body. In Part 1: Chapter 4 "What do I eat doc?", I gave you a list of good fats and bad fats to help make this easier.

Omega-3's help maintain healthy insulin levels, help you avoid excessive inflammation, and help maintain healthy cholesterol levels. I encourage you to purchase good clean omega's free of contaminants such as mercury. Remember, you get what you pay for, so cheap is not always good.

You want to take 1,000-2,000 mg of omega-3 fats per day (should contain a ratio of approximately 300 mg of EPA and 200 mg of DHA), once with breakfast and once with dinner.

For those on a blood thinner such as coumadin or warfarin, there is an interaction between the two and will increase your INR. Please make sure to let your doctor know whenever you are taking any supplement.

Vitamin D3

Vitamin D3 has recently been found to be lacking in a majority of people and at the root of several diseases. In the next chapter I have added one of my three part blog posts for your information.

Magnesium

Diets low in magnesium are associated with increased levels of insulin and we often see magnesium deficiency in diabetics. Magnesium helps glucose enter the cells and turn those calories into energy for the body.

Magnesium also is used for the relief of muscular cramps, spasms and migraines. So I recommend this over nonsteroidal anti-inflammatory (NSAID) like:

• aspirin

• celecoxib (Celebrex)

• diclofenac (Voltaren)

• diflunisal (Dolobid)

• etodolac (Londine)

• ibuprofen (Motrin)

• indomethacin (Indocin)

• ketoprofen (Orudis)

• ketorolac (Toradol)

• nabumetone (Relafen)

• naproxen (Aleve, Naprosyn)

• oxaprozin (Daypro)

• proxicam (Feldene)

• salsalate (Amigesic)

• sulindac (Clinoril)

• tolmetin (Tolectin)

as it is easier on the gut and safer.

Diarrhea is often a sign that you are getting to much magnesium. If this occurs just decrease the dose or switch to magnesium glycinate. You want to avoid magnesium carbonate, sulfate, gluconate, or oxide. These are the cheapest and most common found in supplements plus they are poorly absorbed.

If you tend to be constipated, then I recommend magnesium citrate.

*People with kidney disease or severe heart disease should take magnesium only under a doctor's supervision.

Chapter 3. Vitamin D3

As promised, here is a three part post I did for your understanding regarding Vitamin D3. If you are interested in further information then I warmly invite you to come join us at: www.doctorisabel.com or www.facebook/purelifestyle1.com

Part 1

How is Vitamin D3 produced?

Your skin makes vitamin D3 when it is exposed to a "pinking dose" of sunlight. Depending on your age, how much skin is uncovered and your skin tone, will determine how much vitamin D3 you will make. The darker your skin is, the more sun you need to make enough Vitamin D3.

Sunlight exposure is the main source of vitamin D3 for most people. However, there is no scientifically validated safe level of sun exposure. As a result, it makes recommendations of sun exposure difficult. Why? One needs to weigh the risk of skin damage and skin cancer against the risk of vitamin D3 deficiency.

Children and Vitamin D3:

Dr. Cameron Grant, who is a New Zealand-born pediatrician, has investigated the health of children in New Zealand, and has found the sad truth about their nutritional status. Approximately 14% of New Zealand infants aged 6-23 months are iron deficient; double the rate in Australia, the US, and Europe. And 10% of New Zealand children aged under two have a vitamin D3 deficiency. A quarter of Pacifica children are vitamin D3 deficient. Remember, the darker your skin is, the more sun you need to make enough vitamin D3.

What does that mean? Well, what we are seeing is children having rickets, which can cause bowed legs and knocked knees. Also some children are presenting having convulsions, because their calcium levels are so low. This occurs because they don't have enough vitamin D3 to help absorb the calcium. As a result they have muscle spasms and convulsions.

Regarding pneumonia (which is an infection in the lungs), we are realizing that a vitamin deficiency leads to more pneumonia. So now we know that vitamin D3 maintains a healthy immune function.

Adults and Vitamin D3:

Vitamin D3 is essential for absorbing calcium in the gut. By doing so, it helps reduce the risk of fractures in the elderly.

Below is a list of conditions associated with certain vitamin D3 levels. I show you this because, it is important for you to see what can happen to your health if, your vitamin D3 levels are not in the optimal range.

Levels of vitamin D3 Conditions:

- < 10 ng/ml: Severely deficient

- < 15 ng/ml: Risk of rickets

- < 20 ng/ml: 75% greater risk of colon cancer

< 30 ng/ml Deficient

- Increase calcium loss from bones, osteoporosis

- Poor wound healing

- Increased muscle pain

- Increased joint and back pain

- Greater risk of depression

- Increased diabetes

- Increased schizophrenia

- Increased migraines

- Increased autoimmune disease (lupus, scleroderma)

- Increased allergies

- Increased preeclampsia

- Increased inflammation

- < 34 ng/ml: Twice the risk of heart attacks

- < 36 ng/ml: Increased incidence of high blood pressure

- <100 ng/ml: Increased risk of toxic symptoms (hypercalcemia)

Positives of Higher Levels of Vitamin D3:

- 50 ng/ml: 50% reduction in breast cancer, decreased risk of all solid cancers

- 80-100ng/ml: Slowing of cancer growth in patients with cancer

The Human Warranty:

"We are born with a 70 year warranty, however we never bother to read the instructions. People break down because of owner abuse and neglect, which the usual warranty doesn't cover. Upkeep is the owner's responsibility. That involves a minimum amount of regular use and the right kind of fuel"

- Dr. George Sheehan.

Cardiologist, runner, and writer.

Part 2

I would like to say before we begin, this is so exciting. To be able to give you the information and have you take it on board. All the applause goes to you for implementing this into your life, and your family's life. Ok, here goes.

Below is a little quiz you can take to get an overall idea of your vitamin D3 levels without having to have your blood tested.

Your vitamin D3 quiz

• Do you work indoors?

• Do you hardly ever go outside?

• Do you wear sunblock most of the time?

• Do you have the winter blues, also known as Seasonal Affective Disorder (SAD)?

• Do you suffer from depression?

• Do you have dark skin (any race other than Caucasian)?

• Do you eat small fatty fish such as mackerel, herring, or sardines (the main sources of dietary vitamin D3)?

• Do your muscles feel sore and weak?

• Do your bones feel tender (you can press on your shin bone, and if it hurts, you are low in vitamin D3)?

• Do you have osteoarthritis (Just a reminder, vitamin D3 helps you absorb calcium to make strong bones. Osteoarthritis is a result of low vitamin D3 levels, resulting in weakened bones and thinning of bone structure)?

• Do you have osteoporosis?

• Have you broken more than 2 bones or fractured your hip?

• Do you suffer from mental fogginess or memory loss?

• Do you have autoimmune disease (for example; lupus, multiple sclerosis, scleroderma)?

• Do you have more infections?(like colds, skin or chest infections)

If you scored:Less than 3: then see below on sources of vitamin D34+ : then do the above and see your physician regarding having your vitamin D3 levels checked.

Points about sunblock and vitamin D3:

• We know that vitamin D3 comes from sunlight, however so does skin cancer.

• Without sunblock AND with arms and legs exposed, your skin will make 10,000 to 15,000units of vitamin D3 in one sun exposure, on average. Most people require an additional 2,000 to 5,000 units of vitamin D3 a day

- Sunblock with an SPF of more than 15 blocks 100% of vitamin D3 production in the skin.

My recommendations, as supported by Dr. Mark Hyman, author of The Blood Sugar Solution, are the following; Along side taking a supplement of vitamin D3, the best way to ensure adequate blood levels, is to get 15 minutes of full-body sun exposure between 10 a.m. and 2 p.m., without sunscreen (although we recommend sunscreen on your face). This works only in the summer, so I recommend you take additional vitamin D3 to optimize your level.

Other food sources of vitamin D3 can be found in;

-Mackerel, herring, sardines

-Porcini or shiitake mushrooms

-Cod liver oil.

Part 3

How to check your official levels of vitamin D3?

After reviewing the literature, you want to get your vitamin D3 levels checked with the correct test. Ask to have your 25-OH vitamin D levels checked. The goal is to get your blood levels up to 45-60 ng/ml. I recommend you have your vitamin D3 levels rechecked within 2 weeks to 2 months after starting supplementation and then yearly.

Here are the Vitamin D3 Supplementation Doses

Normal dosing of vitamin D3 depends on your blood levels. Treatment doses (as recommended by The Institute of Functional Medicine) for blood level ranges are:

- <<<10 ng/ml: you want to take 10,000 units per day

- 10-20 ng/ml: you want to take 10,000 units per day

- 20-30 ng/ml: you want to take 8,000 units per day

- 30-40 ng/ml: you want to take 5,000 units per day

- 40-50 ng/dl: you want to take 2,000 units per day

If you are taking a vitamin D3 supplement, adequate calcium and magnesium intake are also required. It is very difficult to get to much vitamin D3. People can take up to 10,000 units per day for 6 months and not have any adverse effects. However, people with sarcoidosis, tuberculosis, Lyme disease, lymphoma, or kidney disease have to be supplemented carefully because of increased risk of their blood calcium level becoming to high.

We have come to the final chapter. To finish off, I always like to have simple guidelines to follow after I have read a book. Below are twelve steps to guide you on the road to your best health, and your permanent weight loss.

Like I say, the best way to break a bad habit, is to replace it with a good one. Be gentle with yourself, and know that failing is all part of the journey. When you do fall, stumble, or just crash and burn...I want you to first forgive yourself, and second dust yourself off, and get back on your road to better health.

12 Steps

1. Eat a **carbohydrate + protein + fat** every 3-4 hours. This helps keep your blood sugar stable.

2. Eat **30 to 60 minutes** upon arising. This gets your metabolism working right away.

3. Eat **low to medium GI foods.** This will keep your insulin from spiking.

4. Avoid all processed foods. Eat only foods your great-great grandmother would recognize.

5. If you are going to cheat, do it in less than one hour. This prevents the insulin spike so you won't store belly fat.

6. No sugar. Just stick to the 1-2 pieces of low GI fruit. I promise you; you won't miss the sugar after a while. Also you will lose weight and have more energy.

7. Drink water. Lots!

8. No food 3 hours before bed. When we don't eat then the glycogen (which is the sugar stored in your liver) is used for the next 6-8 hours. Then after that your body burns fat. You are actually burning fat while you sleep and it's painless. Yahoo!

9. Exercise. Please...

10. Watch what you are saying to yourself. Maintain a positive outlook and be hopeful.

"By altering our attitudes, we can alter our lives."

-Zig Ziglar

" Be careful how you are talking to yourself, because you are listening."

-Lisa M. Hayes

11. Eat good fats.

12. Take your supplements.

One last thought for you. I have given the very best of my heart to you in this book. Now the goal is to incorporate it, to achieve your maximum energy with your best health.

All the applause goes to you, because all I did was coach you. You are the true winners because you implemented these principles into your life and your family's lives.

Your friend,

Isabel

References and Resources <><><><><>

Part One: Your Metabolism and Your Nutrition

Hyman, Dr. Mark. The Blood Sugar Solution. New York. Little, Brown and Co. 2012.

Rubin, Jordan. The Great Physician's Rx for Health and Wellness. Tennessee, Thomas Nelson Inc. 2005.

Foster, Helen. Easy GI Diet. London, Octopus Publishing Group Ltd. 2004.

Kessler, Dr. David. The End of Overeating Taking Control of the Insatiable American Appetite. USA, Rodale Press. 2009.

Lundell, Dr. Dwight. Heart Surgeon Speaks out on What Really Causes Heart Disease. Health Wellness Prevent Disease 01 March 2012.

Part Four: Why Winners win

Hill, Napoleon. The Laws of Success in Sixteen Lessons. Conn. Ralston University Press. 2008.

Part Five: Sugar, Obesity and our future

Dufault R, et al. Mercury from chlor-alkali plants: measured concentrations in food product sugar. Environ Health. 2009 Jan 26;8:2

Bray GA, Nielsen SJ, Popkin BM. Consumption of high-fructose corn syrup in beverages may play a role in the epidemic of obesity. Am J Clin Nutr. 2004 Apr;79(4):537-43. Review.

Swithers SE, Davidson TL. A role for sweet taste: calorie predictive relations in energy regulation by rats. Behav Neurosci. 2008;122 (1):161-73.

Yang Q. Gain weight by "going diet?" Artificial sweeteners, and the neurobiology of sugar cravings. Yale J Biol Med. 2010 June: 83(2):101-108.

Lenoir M, et al. Intense sweetness surpasses cocaine reward. PLoS One. 2007;2 (1):e698.

Ludwig DS. Artificially sweetened beverages: cause for concern. JAMA.2009 Dec 9;302 (22):2477-78.

http://apps.nccd.cdc.gov/DDTSTRS/FactSheet.aspx (National Diabetes Fact 2007).

Part Seven: Putting it all together

Gaby AR. Nutritional Interventions for Muscle Cramps. Integrative Medicine 2007/8, 6(6):20-23.

Rossier P, van Erven S, Wade DT. The effect of magnesium oral therapy on spasticity in a patient with multiple sclerosis. European Jouranal of Neurology 2000, 7(6): 741-744.

Braun L & Cohen M, Chromium, Herbs and Natural Supplements: An evidence-based guide 3rd Edition Sydney, Elsevier, 2010, pp. 320=326.

Facchinetti F, et al, Magnesium prophylaxis of menstral migraine: effects on intracellular magnesium Headache, 1991: 31:298-301.

Peikert A, et al Prophylaxis of migraine with oral magnesium: results from a prospective, multi-center, palcebo-controlled and double-blind randomized study. Cephalalgia, 196:16:257-263.

Sun-Edelstein C and Mauskop A, Role of magnesium in the pathogenesis and treatment of migraine. Expert Review of Neurotherapeutics, 2009; 9(3):369.

Braun L, Cohen M. Zinc, Herbs and Natural Supplements;an evidence based guide; Elsevier Australia 2010, pp. 1037-1054.

Braun L, Cohen M. Selenium-Herbs, and Natural Supplements; an evidence based guide; Elsevier Australia 2010, pp. 844-56.

Butterworth R. Chapter 23: Thiamine. In Shils ME, et al (Eds), Modern Nutrition in Health and Disease 10th Edition, Philadelphia, Lippincott Williams and Wilkins 2006: pp. 426-433.

Homocysteine Lowering Trialists Collaboration. Dose-dependent effects of folic acid on blood concentrations of homocysteine: a meta analysis of the randomized trials. Am J Clin Nutr 2005; 82(4): 806-12.

The Blood Sugar Solution by Mark Hyman, MD p.75-77.

Nikooyeh B, et al. Daily consumption of vitamin D- or vitamin D + calcium-fortified yogurt drink improved glycemin control in patients with type 2 diabetes: a randomized clinical trial. Am J Clin Nutr. 2011 Apr; 93(4):764-71.

The Vitamin D Factor by Jennifer Bowden. New Zealand Listener. April 21, 2012. Issue 3754

Institute of Functional Medicine:

Dietary Supplement Fact Sheet: Vitamin D. Office of Dietary Supplements (ODS). National Institutes of Health (NIH). Retrieved 2010-04 11.b.Cedric F. Garland, Dr PH, FACE, Edward D. Gorham, MPH, PhD, Sharif B. Mohr, MPH, Frank C. Garland, PhD. Vitamin D for cancer prevention: Global perspective. Annals of Epidemiology. Volume 19, Issue 7, Pages 468-483 (July 2009).c.P. Lips, D. Hosking, K. Lippuner, J. M. Norquist, L. Wehren, G. Maalouf, S. Ragi-Eis, J. Chandler. The prevalence of vitamin D inadequacy amongst women with osteoporosis: an international epidemiological investigation. Volume 260, Issue 3, pages 245–254, September 2006d.Siegfried Segaer. Vitamin D regulation of cathelicidin in the skin: Toward a renaissance of vitamin D in Dermatology? Journal of Investigative Dermatology (2008) 128, 773–775. doi:10.1038/jid.2008.35e.Plotnikoff GA, Quigley JM. Prevalence of severe hypovitaminosis D in patients with persistent, nonspecific musculoskeletal pain. Mayo Clin Proc. 2003;78(12):1463-1470.f. Al Faraj, Saud MD; Al Mutairi, Khalaf MD. Vitamin D deficiency and chronic low back pain in Saudi Arabia. Spine:15 January 2003 - Volume 28 - Issue 2 - pp 177-179.g.Armstrong, D.; Meenagh, G.; Bickle, I.; Lee, A.; Curran, E.; Finch, M Vitamin D deficiency is associated with anxiety and depression in fibromyalgia. Clinical Rheumatology. Volume 26, Number 4, 551-554, DOI: 10.1007/s10067-006-0348-5h. Mathieu C, Gysemans C, Giulietti A, Bouillon R. Vitamin D and diabetes. Diabetologia. 2006 Jan;49(1):217-8.i. Mackay-Sim A, Féron F, Eyles D, Burne T, McGrath J. Schizophrenia, vitamin D, and brain development. Int Rev Neurobiol. 2004;59:351-80.j. Vitamin D Deficiency Common in Patients with Chronic Migraine. http://www.medscape.com/viewarticle/577151k. Ginanjar E, Sumariyono, Setiati S, Setiyohadi B. Vitamin D and autoimmune disease. Acta Med Indones. 2007 Jul-Sep;39(3):133-41.l. Lisa M. Bodnar, Janet M. Catov, Hyagriv N. Simhan, Michael F. Holick, Robert W. Powers and James M. Roberts. Maternal vitamin D deficiency increases the risk of preeclampsia. The Journal of Clinical Endocrinology & Metabolism Vol. 92, No. 9 3517-3522m.Int J Epidemiol. 1990 Sep;19(3):559-63. Myocardial infarction is inversely associated with plasma 25-hydroxyvitamin D3 levels: a community-based study. Scragg R, Jackson R, Holdaway IM, Lim T, Beaglehole R. Department of Community Health, University of Auckland , New Zealand.n. Li YC, Kong J, Wei M, Chen ZF, Liu SQ, Cao LP. 1,25-Dihydroxyvitamin D(3) is a negative endocrine regulator of the renin-angiotensin system. J Clin Invest. 2002;110(2):229-238.o. Ramagopalan SV, Maugeri NJ, Handunnetthi L, Lincoln MR, Orton S-M, et al. (2009) Expression of the multiple sclerosis-associated MHC Class II Allele HLA-DRB1*1501 Is regulated by vitamin D. PLoS Genet 5(2): e1000369. doi:10.1371/journal.pgen.1000369p. Anderson L, Cotterchio M, Vieth R, Knight J. Vitamin D and calcium intakes and breast cancer risk I npre- and postmenopausal women. Am J Clin Nutr 2010; 91(6): 1699-1701.q.Garland CF, Gorham ED, Mohr SB, et al. Vitamin D and prevention of breast cancer: Pooled analysis. J Steroid Biochem Mol Biol 2007;103:708–11.r.Bruce W Hollis and Carol L Wagner. Assessment of dietary vitamin D requirements during pregnancy and lactation. American Journal of Clinical Nutrition, Vol. 79, No. 5, 717-726, May 2004

About the Author <><><><>

Dr. Isabel Bertran-Hunsinger is a Cuban-American, now living on the North Island of New Zealand. She moved there from USA to NZ to offer the family a different way of life, and yes, she has gotten that. Her girls even have the gorgeous Kiwi accent. She loves to do anything that keeps her fitness going, and Isabel enjoys biking, walking, trekking and training at the Gym. Her husband, Michael, and Isabel have been in love (yes, marriage!) for 33 years and are excited about reaching 100 years young, together. Isabel thoroughly loves her walk with God, as she says, "my Christianity is the backbone of my life."

Dr. Isabel believes that you are your best doctor, you just need a health coach to guide you. The goal is to have fun while we learn together the four principles of the Dr. Isabel platform; HEAL; Health, Education, Attitude and Leadership.

Dr. Isabel offers health coaching to clients all over the World. She currently has a limited number of spaces available for 1×1 consultations via Skype, or other media sources. Contact her via email or Skype to set-up a Free initial consultation. Please note; Dr. Isabel is not to replace your physician. Your consultation with her as a Healthy Lifestyle Coach, is alongside your doctor to empower your health, so you can live "Life to the Max".

Isabel Bertran-Hunsinger M.D. (aka Dr.Isabel)University Of Colorado Medical School 1991

Southern Colorado Family Practice Residency 1995

Fellow of the Royal New Zealand College of General Practice 2005

Member of the Institute of Functional Medicine

Dr. Isabel Speaking Availability <><><><>

   Dr. Isabel is available to speak for corporate functions, business team-building, and public groups. Your PureLifestyle Plan, Healthy Lifestyle Program, would be an excellent way to improve productivity on a personal and business team level. We can provide personalized assessment programs for you and your staff. A healthy team engages better around company goals, and Team members are mentally present. This leads to greater productivity, which leads to profits. Check the "contact Dr.Isabel" page for contact information. To have your team, or you personally, "Living Life to the Max", give Isabel a call, Skype, or e-mail today.

Whether you want a health coach, inspirational speaker, or guidance on natural supplements. Dr. Isabel can be contacted via Skype, Facebook, Twitter or Email. Please refer to the details below:

Skype: *isabel.hunsinger*

Facebook: *https://www.facebook.com/purelifestyle1*

Twitter: *https://twitter.com/purelifestyle1*

Website/Blog: www.doctorisabel.co.nz

Check www.doctorisabel.co.nz for the upcoming date of "Your PureLifestyle Cleanse" for your start to permanent weight loss.

www.ingramcontent.com/pod-product-compliance
Lightning Source LLC
Chambersburg PA
CBHW022118280326
41933CB00007B/445